POCKET GUIDE FOR

# CARDIAC
# ELECTROPHYSIOLOGY

**JOHN D. HUMMEL, MD**
M__ C_____logy Consultants
C_____

**S_____ _____LEISCH, MD**
_____logy Consultants

**JOA___ ____LON, RN, CCRN**
___t Hospital

**___ _____ COMPANY**
_____rt Brace & Company
___on • Toronto • Montreal • Sydney • Tokyo

**W.B. SAUNDERS COMPANY**

*A Division of Harcourt Brace & Company*

The Curtis Center
Independence Square West
Philadelphia, Pennsylvania 19106

---

**Library of Congress Cataloging-in-Publication Data**

Hummel, John D.
    Pocket guide for a cardiac electrophysiology / John D. Hummel, Steven Jack Kalbfleisch, Joanne M. Dillon.
      p.  cm.
    ISBN 0–7216–7369–4
    1. Electrocardiography Handbooks, manuals, etc.  2. Heart—Electric properties Handbooks, manuals, etc.
  3. Electrophysiology Handbooks, manuals, etc.  I. Kalbfleisch, Steven Jack.  II. Dillon, Joanne M.  III. Title.
    [DNLM: 1. Electrophysiology Handbooks.  2. Heart—physiology handbooks.  WG 39 H925p 2000]
  RC683.5.E5H79  2000
  616.1′207547—dc21
  DNLM/DLC                                     99–23883

---

POCKET GUIDE FOR CARDIAC ELECTROPHYSIOLOGY        ISBN 0–7216–7369–4

Printed in the United States of America

Last digit is the print number:    9    8    7    6    5    4    3    2    1

# PREFACE

Clinical cardiac electrophysiology has evolved from a field of primarily diagnostic evaluation of arrhythmias to one in which intervention, in the form of catheter ablation or device implantation, often forms the mainstay of therapy. These changes have led to an increase in the demand for electrophysiologic laboratories and knowledgeable associated personnel.

In our institution, we observed that each new staff member had the tendency to piece together a "notebook." Contained in this was critical information regarding the procedures performed in the lab and the information needed to work effectively and efficiently with the electrophysiologist. The purpose of this text is to obliverate the need for such a "notebook" and to provide nurses, technicians, medical students, and cardiology fellows with a compact and concise reference that can be used day to day to help guide one through the myriad of procedures being performed in the electrophysiology laboratory. The chapters are designed to allow one to quickly develop an idea of what will be happening in an upcoming procedure, and to understand why certain steps are undertaken during the procedures.

The book is based upon the approach taken by electrophysiologists and nurses in a high volume electrophysiology center where both clinical and research procedures are performed. We would like to thank the electrophysiology nurses at Riverside Methodist Hospitals who work with us on a daily basis. We would also like to thank Judy Annis for her assistance with manuscript preparation.

*John D. Hummel, M.D.*
*Steven J. Kalbfleisch, M.D.*
*Joanne M. Dillon, R.N.*

# CONTENTS

# CHAPTER 1

# ELECTROPHYSIOLOGY LABORATORY SET-UP

There are numerous diagnostic tests and therapeutic interventions for evaluating and treating patients with known or suspected cardiac arrhythmias and syncope. Invasive procedures usually require the use of fluoroscopy. Noninvasive procedures do not require the use of fluoroscopy and can be done in a non-fluoroscopy laboratory. This strategy maximizes the availability of the fluoroscopy laboratory for invasive procedures. The laboratories needed to perform these tests and interventions are shown in Table 1–1.

## ELECTROPHYSIOLOGY LABORATORY EQUIPMENT

The electrophysiology study is a type of heart catheterization that requires much of the same equipment found in a general catheterization laboratory. Additional equipment is specifically required for assessing the cardiac electrical system. The equipment necessary for an electrophysiology laboratory is listed in Chart 1–1.

| **Table 1-1** | LABORATORY TYPE AND TESTING REQUIRED FOR EVALUATING CARDIAC ARRHYTHMIAS AND SYNCOPE |
|---|---|
| Invasive laboratory | Noninvasive laboratory |
|   Electrophysiology study |   Tilt table testing |
|   Radiofrequency catheter ablation |   Cardioversion |
|   Pacemaker implantation |   Defibrillator testing |
|   Defibrillator implantation | |

The fluoroscopy unit must have an image intensifier and be capable of providing views in multiple planes. The radiographic table should be able to move easily into multiple positions guided by the person placing and manipulating the catheters. A cardiac stimulator, necessary for pacing the heart, should have the capability of sensing cardiac events and delivering pacing stimuli at programmable intervals.

The multichannel data acquisition system should have such features as the ability to record at different speeds from 25 to 500 mm/sec and signal filtering capabilities for both surface and intracardiac channels. It should be able to record three or four surface electrocardiograms (ECGs) with multiple intracardiac electrograms. Ideally, the system has pressure monitoring capability and a storage medium such as an optical disk.

Two waveform monitors are recommended. One is located near the cardiac stimulator and the other near the fluoroscopy table for ease of viewing during catheter manipulation. Simultaneous 12-lead ECG recordings can be obtained from a free-standing device or as a feature of the data acquisition system.

## Chart 1-1
### ELECTROPHYSIOLOGY LABORATORY EQUIPMENT

- Fluoroscopy unit
- Radiographic table
- Cardiac stimulator
- Multichannel data acquisition system
- 12-Lead electrocardiography (ECG)
- ECG display screens (oscilloscopes)
- Multichannel lead switching box
- Resuscitation/emergency equipment
- Pulse oximetry
- Invasive or noninvasive blood pressure monitor
- Intravenous infusion pump
- Radiofrequency lesion generator
- Electrosurgical cautery
- Pacemaker lead analyzer (PSA)
- Implantable device programmers

The multichannel lead switching box should have multiple catheter input capability and the ability to switch each catheter between pacing and recording. The layout for equipment specific to the electrophysiology laboratory is shown in Figure 1–1.

Resuscitation equipment necessary in the laboratory includes two defibrillators, one serving as backup in the event that the other fails. The defibrillators should have pacing capability and be able to deliver defibrillation through "hands-free" pads or standard paddles. Other emergency items required are a temporary pacing unit, suction equipment, oxygen supplementation equipment, and intubation apparatus.

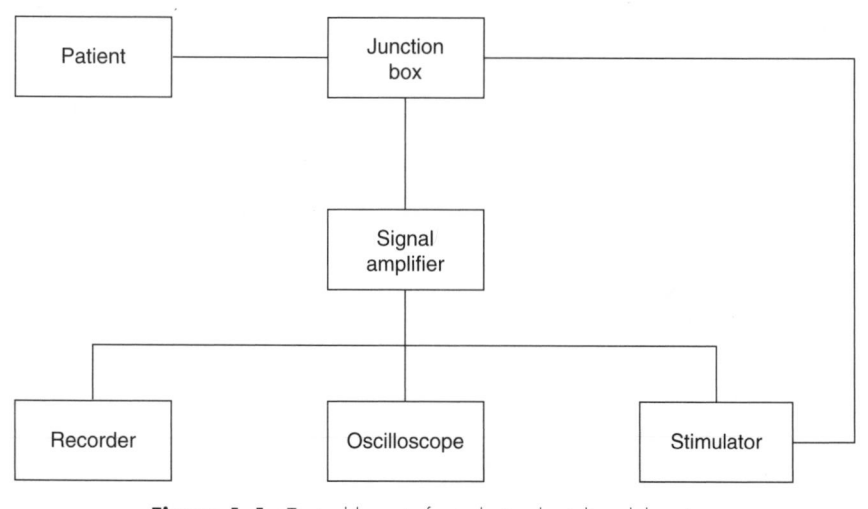

**Figure 1–1 •** Typical layout of an electrophysiology laboratory.

Pulse oximetry must be available to monitor the patient's response to conscious sedation. $CO_2$ monitoring is beneficial when assessing patients who are in deep sedation for extended periods. Invasive or noninvasive blood pressure monitoring is required to monitor hemodynamic status.

An intravenous infusion pump must be available for continuous administration of medications during electrophysiology procedures. The radiofrequency lesion generator is necessary if catheter ablation procedures are to be performed. Electrosurgical cautery is necessary to control hemostasis during insertion of implantable devices. A pacemaker lead analyzer system (PSA) should be available for determining proper lead placement during pacemaker and defibrillator implantation. Implantable device programmers for both pacemakers and internal cardiac defibrillators are available from the manufacturers and should be located in close proximity to the laboratory to allow convenient device programming.

## EQUIPMENT MAINTENANCE

Electrophysiology (EP) laboratory equipment requires careful maintenance. All new equipment should be inspected and labeled by the biomedical engineering department prior to usage. Existing equipment is inspected at intervals according to the institution's protocol. Emergency equipment, such as defibrillators, is tested by EP laboratory staff on a regular basis as required by regulatory standards. Documentation records must be maintained.

## MINIMIZING RECORDING INTERFERENCE

Electrical interference may create artifacts, rendering cardiac recordings that are difficult to interpret. A number of methods, listed in Chart 1–2, can be employed to minimize that likelihood.

 **Chart 1-2**
METHODS USED TO MINIMIZE RECORDING ARTIFACTS

- Ground equipment properly
- Isolate electrophysiology laboratory electrical supply source
- Shield and suspend wires and cables
- Use recording apparatus notch filters
- Utilize proper skin preparation for surface electrodes
- Address patient tremor with warm blankets and medications

- Avoid use of extension cords
- Unplug any unnecessary electrical equipment
- Secure electrical equipment cables tightly into wall plug
- Move electrical equipment cables to different circuits should interference occur
- Utilize biomedical engineering resources to assist in initial laboratory setup and troubleshoot problems as they occur

## ELECTROPHYSIOLOGY LABORATORY SUPPLIES

Supplies in the EP laboratory consist of those needed for patient preparation and for obtaining vascular access. Other items necessary are electrode catheters, medications, and documentation records.

Supplies required to prepare the patient for EP procedures are listed in Chart 1–3. A disposable sterile procedure pack is generally used for obtaining vascular access. The items most commonly used for this purpose are listed in Chart 1–4.

During EP studies introducers, sheaths, electrode catheters, and sterile catheter connecting cables are added to the tray once venous access is established. The manufacturer and the type and number of catheters used during a procedure depends on electrophysiologist's preference.

---

 **Chart 1-3**
PATIENT PROCEDURE PREPARATION SUPPLIES

- Pacing/defibrillation electrodes
- ECG electrodes
- Blood pressure cuff
- Reusable or disposable pulse oximetry sensor

- Disposable razors
- Wedge cushion to elevate feet if radiography table does not have a Trendelenburg feature

---

**Chart 1–4**
DISPOSABLE STERILE VENOUS ACCESS INSTRUMENTATION PACK CONTENTS

- Sponges
- Antimicrobial scrub solution, local anesthetic agent, and heparinized saline
- Solution containers
- Seldinger or single-entry needle for access

- Needles and syringes
- Sponges
- Sterile drapes
- Hemostats
- Cook or Potts needle

A different type of sterile procedure pack is used for pacemaker and defibrillator implantation. In addition to the availability of a surgical instrument tray, the items listed in Chart 1–5 are commonly used during device implantation and are included or added to the sterile pack. Additional supplies required for the EP laboratory are intravenous infusion pumps and a patient transfer device.

## STOCK MEDICATIONS

Stock medications for the EP laboratory should be easily accessible. Commonly used medications are listed in Chart 1–6.

## Chart 1-5
### DISPOSABLE STERILE PACEMAKER PACK CONTENTS

- Large basin for sterile saline
- Local anesthetic agent
- Solution containers
- Large irrigation syringe
- Suction tubing
- Bovie pen
- Bovie tip cleaner
- Syringes and needles
- Sponges
- Pacemaker drape
- Scalpel
- Suture
- Introducers
- Steri-Strips™
- Gowns
- Gloves
- Towels

## Chart 1-6
### STOCK MEDICATIONS FOR THE ELECTROPHYSIOLOGY LABORATORY

- Sedation/analgesia agents: midazolam (Versed), propofol, fentanyl, diphenhydramine (Benadryl), droperidol
- Reversal agents: naloxone (Narcan) and flumazenil (Romazicon)
- Antiemetics
- Atropine
- Isoproterenol
- Adenosine
- Epinephrine
- Verapamil
- Aspirin
- Procainamide

## LABORATORY PERSONNEL REQUIREMENTS

Personnel requirements for the EP laboratory depend on the complexity and risks of the procedure, the baseline physical condition of the patient, the amount of sedation given, and staff training. State laws and credentialing organizations may mandate that staff with certain expertise be present during the procedure. Other than the electrophysiologist, the staff may consist of a mix of registered nurses, radiation technologists, and technicians.

## INFECTION CONTROL AND ELECTRICAL AND RADIATION SAFETY

Infection control and electrical and radiation safety are high priority issues in the EP laboratory. Strategies used to decrease risks to the patient and staff are listed in Charts 1–7, 1–8, and 1–9.

## LABORATORY EFFICIENCY

Scheduling practices affect the efficiency of the laboratory. It is important to schedule procedures in a manner that promotes optimal utilization of invasive laboratory time. Although each institution must develop its own unique system, several strategies may be helpful when developing a more predictable scheduling method (Chart 1–10).

Many patient processing and staff issues affect laboratory operations. The capacity of the laboratory is diminished when nonessential tasks are performed inside rather than outside the invasive laboratory.

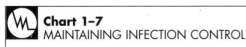

**Chart 1-7**
MAINTAINING INFECTION CONTROL

- Practice universal precautions
- Wash hands before and after procedures
- Properly sterilize and store instruments and supplies
- Minimize traffic flow in electrophysiology (EP) laboratory
- Administer prophylactic antibiotic therapy for device implantation
- Maintain proper temperature, humidity, state or regulatory required air exchange in laboratory
- Decontaminate EP laboratory for device implantation according to the institution's surgery room standards
- Isolate patient incision or puncture site with sterile draping
- Properly dispose of sharps and needles
- Wear protective barrier during high risk procedures
- Maintain separate clean storage and decontamination areas

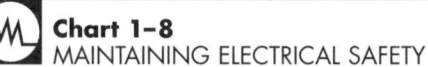

### Chart 1-8
#### MAINTAINING ELECTRICAL SAFETY

- Turn off operated equipment prior to disconnecting from wall outlet
- Remove, label "malfunctioning," and have repaired any dropped, damaged, or malfunctioning equipment
- Keep patient area clean and dry
- Do not permit any nonstandard equipment repairs

- Use properly grounded equipment and hospital grade power cords
- Inspect power cords for damage or wear
- Cover equipment controls with faceplates
- Report any suspected problem to the bioengineering department

**Chart 1-9**
MAINTAINING RADIATION SAFETY

- Wear encircling lead aprons and thyroid shields
- Determine if female patients are pregnant
- Wear radiation safety badge and monitor staff exposure
- Alert staff before activating fluoroscopy
- Shield electrophysiology laboratory and walls with lead lining

- Inspect fluoroscopy equipment at intervals mandated by state/federal guidelines
- Post signs to indicate "x-ray in use"
- Maintain greatest possible distance from the radiation field
- Maintain image intensifier in a position that minimizes exposure to the patient and staff

**Chart 1-10**
OPTIMAL SCHEDULING STRATEGIES

- Monitor individual physician or group procedure-times; schedule procedures based on known individual average procedure times
- Monitor individual physician or group monthly volume percentages on a quarterly basis; block out weekly physician or group times based on average volume percentages; revise on a regular basis
- "Build in" time to accommodate unanticipated events (i.e., procedure duration longer than planned)

Moreover, the laboratory may be underutilized when staff who are qualified to assist with invasive procedures are spending time performing tasks that can be undertaken by ancillary support staff. There are many opportunities to increase laboratory capacity and efficiency, as suggested in Chart 1–11.

---

 **Chart 1-11**
### STRATEGIES TO IMPROVE PATIENT FLOW

- Perform noninvasive tests and procedures near but not in the electrophysiology (EP) laboratory.
- Tilt table testing can be performed by qualified staff without the physician present so long as the physician is in an adjacent area.
- Nondirect patient care tasks should be performed by nonclinical staff (e.g., scheduling, patient transfers, stocking the laboratory).
- Patient procedure preparation and depreparation can be done in an area adjacent to the EP laboratory, such as in a holding area.
- Dedicated housekeeping and transport personnel improve the laboratory turnover time.

---

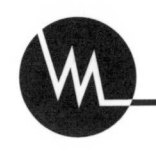

# CHAPTER 2

# BASIC PRINCIPLES OF THE ELECTROPHYSIOLOGY STUDY

The electrophysiology (EP) study is an invasive procedure in which intracardiac electrode catheters are used to evaluate a broad spectrum of cardiac arrhythmias. It can evaluate the function of the sinus node, atrioventricular (AV) node, and His-Purkinje system; and it can determine if inducible supraventricular or ventricular arrhythmias are present.

## INDICATIONS

The indications for EP studies have been summarized in an ACC/AHA Task Force report (published in the *Journal of American College of Cardiology*, 1989). The indications were divided into three classes that defined the clinical necessity of the procedure: Class I definitely substantiates the need for study; class II suggests that the study is probably or possibly indicated; class III suggests that the study is not indicated, as it would not provide useful information. The ACC/AHA Task Force guidelines for EP studies are summarized in Chart 2–1.

### Chart 2-1
### ACC/AHA TASK FORCE REPORT ON GUIDELINES FOR CLINICAL INTRACARDIAC ELECTROPHYSIOLOGY STUDIES

Class I indications: electrophysiology study indicated

- Symptomatic patients with suspected sinus node dysfunction or His-Purkinje block not apparent on electrocardiogram (ECG)
- Patients with a pacemaker for heart block with suspected ventricular arrhythmias as a cause of their symptoms
- Patients with bundle branch block: suspected ventricular arrhythmias as a cause of their symptoms
- Patients not tolerating or not responding to medications for narrow QRS tachycardia in whom the study would alter therapy
- Patients with narrow QRS tachycardia preferring ablative therapy
- Patients with sustained wide QRS complex tachycardias
- Patients with an accessory pathway tachycardia that is symptomatic and may require ablative therapy

*continues*

### Chart 2-1
#### ACC/AHA TASK FORCE REPORT ON GUIDELINES FOR CLINICAL INTRACARDIAC ELECTROPHYSIOLOGY STUDIES *(Continued)*

- Patients with unexplained syncope and known structural heart disease
- Patients surviving cardiac arrest without Q wave myocardial infarction or surviving cardiac arrest occurring >48 hours after acute myocardial infarction
- Patients with palpitations and documented inappropriately rapid pulse rates without apparent cause
- Patients who are candidates for implantation of an electrical device to treat their arrhythmias or have an implanted device and require therapy changes that may alter the safety or efficacy of their device
- Patients who may be candidates for antiarrhythmic surgery or ablation
- Patients who have had antiarrhythmic medication, surgery, or ablation to evaluate the efficacy of current and future therapy

Class II indications: electrophysiology study may be indicated
- Patients with sinus node dysfunction to exclude other arrhythmic causes or assess the severity or mechanism of dysfunction and drug response to direct therapy
- Patients with second or third degree atrioventricular block to determine the site or mechanism of the block in order to direct therapy

- Symptomatic patients with bundle branch block to assess the site and severity of the conduction delay in order to direct therapy and evaluate prognosis
- Asymptomatic patients with ECG evidence of Wolff-Parkinson-White syndrome to evaluate the accessory pathway in high risk activities, a family history of premature sudden death, or unexplained syncope
- Patients with premature ventricular complexes and unexplained presyncope or syncope
- Patients with clinically significant cardiac palpitations thought to be of cardiac origin but not documented by noninvasive testing in order to diagnose, treat, and assess prognosis
- Risk stratify postmyocardial infarction patients with reduced left ventricular function having frequent premature ventricular contractions, nonsustained ventricular tachycardia, or both, particularly if the signal-averaged ECG shows the presence of late potentials

Class III indications: electrophysiology study is not indicated

- Symptomatic patients with sinus node dysfunction with ECG documentation of a brady-arrhythmia cause
- Asymptomatic patients with bradyarrhythmia during sleep
- Patients with congenital QT prolongation or with acquired prolonged QT syndrome with symptoms related to an identifiable cause or mechanism
- Patients with a known cause of syncope
- Patients with cardiac arrest occurring only within the first 48 hours of acute myocardial infarction

## POTENTIAL RISKS AND COMPLICATIONS

Electrophysiology testing is associated with low mortality and morbidity. In general, the risks are similar to those posed by standard cardiac catheterization. The complications associated with EP studies depend on the access site used and are listed in Chart 2–2.

## CONTRAINDICATIONS

There are few contraindications to EP testing. In general, most of the contraindications are related to the potential inability to maintain hemostasis, clinical stability, and infection control; there is also a minimal risk of thrombosis. Specific contraindications to electrophysiology testing are listed in Chart 2–3.

---

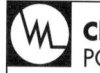

**Chart 2–2**
POTENTIAL RISKS AND COMPLICATIONS OF ELECTROPHYSIOLOGY STUDIES

- Hypotension
- Hematoma
- Hemorrhage

- Vascular injury
- Thrombophlebitis
- Systemic emboli

- Acute cardiac tamponade
- Pneumothorax
- Death

---

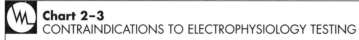

**Chart 2-3**
CONTRAINDICATIONS TO ELECTROPHYSIOLOGY TESTING

- Bleeding disorder
- Unstable angina
- Uncontrolled congestive heart failure
- Uncooperative patient
- Severe peripheral vascular disease
- Valvular or subvalvular stenosis (left ventricular access)
- Thrombophlebitis (femoral access)
- Groin infection
- Bilateral amputee (femoral access)

## ELECTROPHYSIOLOGY CATHETERS

Electrophysiology catheters consist of insulated wires attached to electrodes at the distal tip of the catheter. Once the catheter is inserted into the heart, these electrodes impinge on the endocardial surface. The proximal end of the catheter is connected to external devices that record or allow delivery of pacing stimuli—the two essential functions of EP studies.

Catheter selection is usually a matter of physician preference. Adult EP catheters range in size from 5F to 7F. It is generally recommended that the sheath introducers be 1F larger than the catheter.

The quadripolar (four electrode) catheter is the one most commonly used. It has two electrodes for monitoring and two for pacing. The distal portion of the catheter may have a special bend or curve that facilitates placement in certain areas of the heart. The spacing between electrodes ranges from 2.5 to 10.0

mm. Distal electrode size varies from 2 to 8 mm. Ablative procedures typically employ distal electrodes larger than 4 mm. Figure 2–1 shows a quadripolar catheter.

## CATHETER INSERTION SITES AND LOCATIONS

Selection of a catheter access site for an EP study depends on patient accessibility and physician preference. Most EP studies are performed by accessing the right femoral vein. Figure 2–2 shows the most common access sites. Generally, a catheter is positioned in the high right atrium, in the His bundle position, and in the right ventricular apex or outflow tract. Figure 2–3 shows typical catheter placement positions during EP studies. A summary of the more commonly desired electrograms, usual access sites, and fluoroscopic descriptions of catheter location are provided in Table 2–1.

On occasion, pacing and recording in the left atrium or ventricle is necessary. Several techniques have been developed to preclude accessing the arterial system or facilitate placement of catheters in the left or arterial side of the heart. These techniques are discussed below.

### Coronary Os

A catheter placed in the coronary os is capable of recording left atrial and left ventricular electrograms because the coronary sinus lies in the atrioventricular (AV) groove between the left atrium and left ventricle. The benefit of this technique is avoidance of arterial access. Pacing the left ventricle with this approach, however, is unreliable. Figure 2–4 shows placement of a catheter in the coronary sinus.

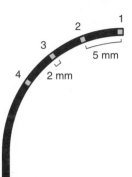

**Figure 2-1 •** Quadripolar catheter. The electrodes are numbered 1 through 4. The distal tip is number 1. The number and spacing of electrodes varies, depending on the intended purpose of the catheter.

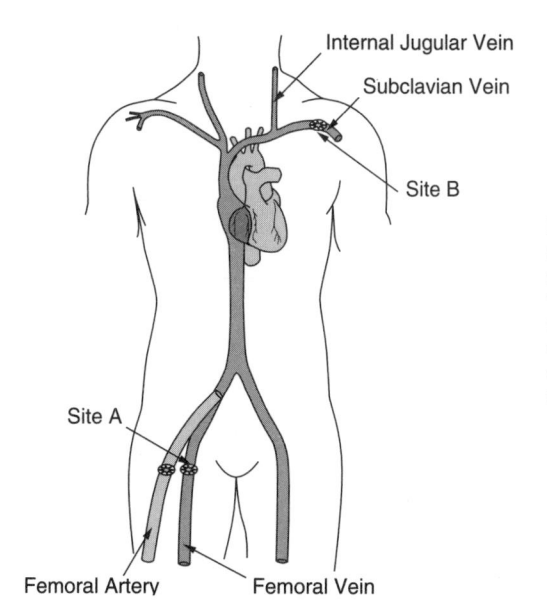

Internal Jugular Vein

Subclavian Vein

Site B

Site A

Femoral Artery

Femoral Vein

**Figure 2-2 •** Commonly used vascular access sites for electrophysiology (EP)-related procedures. Site A (right femoral vein) is the typical access site for EP/ablation procedures. Site B (subclavian vein) is the usual site for pacemaker and nonthoracotomy internal cardiac defibrillators.

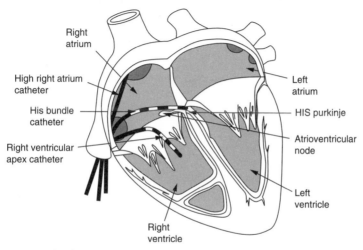

**Figure 2-3** • Typical catheter placement sites during an electrophysiology study. One catheter is placed in the high right atrium, one in the His bundle position, and one at the right ventricular apex or outflow tract.

| **Table 2-1** CATHETER APPROACH AND FLUOROSCOPIC DESCRIPTION FOR ELECTROPHYSIOLOGY STUDIES | | |
|---|---|---|
| **SITE OF ELECTROGRAM** | **ACCESS SITE** | **FLUOROSCOPIC DESCRIPTION** |
| Right atrium | Right femoral vein | Right atrium, high lateral wall superior vena cava junction |
| His bundle | Right femoral vein | Posterior aspect of tricuspid valve |
| Coronary sinus | Internal jugular, subclavian vein, or right femoral vein | Coronary sinus os (posterior and inferior to tricuspid valve) |
| Right ventricle | Right femoral vein | Right ventricle and ventricular outflow tract |
| Left atrium | Right femoral vein | Left atrium via atrial septal defect or patent foramen ovale |
| | Right femoral vein | Left atrium via transseptal approach (needle puncture of atrial septum) |
| | Right femoral artery | Left atrium via mitral valve |
| Left ventricle | Right femoral artery | Left ventricle via aortic valve |

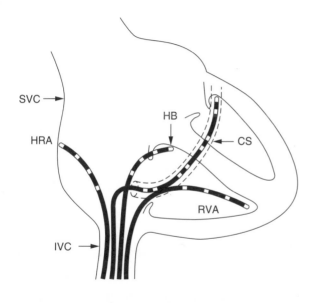

**Figure 2-4** • Catheter placement in the coronary sinus (CS). The coronary sinus lies in the AV sulcus between the left atrium and the left ventricle, allowing electrode catheter recording from the left atrium and left ventricle. The electrode catheter is introduced via the femoral vein. SVC, IVC = superior and inferior vena cava; HRA = high right atrium; HB = His bundle; RVA = right ventricular apex.

## Foramen Ovale

Two approaches are used to access the left atrium: (1) crossing the atrial septum and (2) from a femoral vein. One method utilizes a patent foramen ovale, which is present in only a small percentage of patients. This small, clinically irrelevant opening sometimes permits direct entry of the catheter from the right atrium into the left atrium.

### Transseptal Approach

The transseptal approach provides left atrial access. Additional supplies needed for a transseptal puncture include a Brockenbrough needle and stylet and a Brockenbrough catheter or Mullins sheath. The technique involves induction of a sheath from the right femoral vein. The atrial septum is then punctured using a transseptal needle, and the sheath is advanced to the left atrium. The catheter is advanced through the sheath once heparinization is achieved. Transseptal puncture of the atrial septum is shown in Figure 2–5.

### Retrograde Approach

Two other techniques for approaching the left side of the heart involve access through the right femoral artery. The retrograde approach provides left ventricular access by advancing the catheter retrogradely across the aortic valve into the left ventricle. The left atrium can also be approached directly by retrograde catheterization from the left ventricle across the mitral valve.

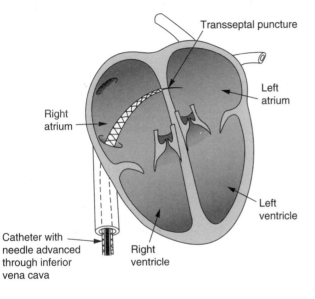

Right atrium

Transseptal puncture

Left atrium

Catheter with needle advanced through inferior vena cava

Right ventricle

Left ventricle

**Figure 2–5 •** Transseptal catheter crossing the atrial septum and lying in the left atrium.

## BASIC ELECTROPHYSIOLOGY STUDY

The basic EP study consists of measuring baseline conduction intervals and evaluating the patient's response to programmed electrical stimulation.

### Baseline Intervals

Once the catheters are in place, various electrode pairs are set up for pacing and recording. Typically, three or four electrocardiographic (ECG) surface lead recordings and intracardiac electrograms from each electrode catheter placed are displayed on the oscilloscopes. An example of a typical baseline EP study recording is shown in Figure 2–6.

Baseline conduction intervals are determined at the beginning of the study. The baseline measurement protocol involves recording and measuring surface ECG and intracardiac electrogram conduction intervals. Measurements of these intervals are shown in Figure 2–7.

The His bundle electrogram provides useful information about the conduction velocity of the AV node. Conduction velocity is the speed of conduction of an electrical impulse across the heart. The His bundle catheter, once positioned, records electrical activity of the low right atrium, AV node, His bundle, and a portion of the right ventricle. The AH interval represents the conduction time through the AV node to the His bundle. This interval may vary up to 20 ms during a single study as it is affected by the patient's autonomic tone. The HV interval represents conduction time through the His-Purkinje system. This interval is

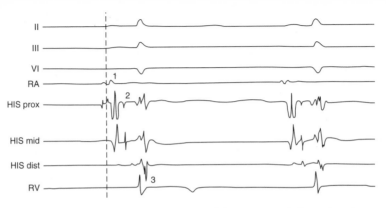

**Figure 2-6** • Surface and intracardiac recordings obtained during a typical electrophysiology study. Surface recordings are leads II, III, and V₁. Intracardiac recordings are from the right atrium (RA), His bundle (proximal, mid, and distal recordings), and right ventricle (RV). This is an example or an intracardiac recording of sinus conduction. The diagnosis of sinus rhythm is confirmed by the sequence of intracardiac electrical activity. The earliest electrical activity is recorded from the RA catheter (1), which is expected because the SA node initiates sinus rhythm. Subsequently, conduction proceeds to the AV node (2) and through the His bundle (3) to the RV.

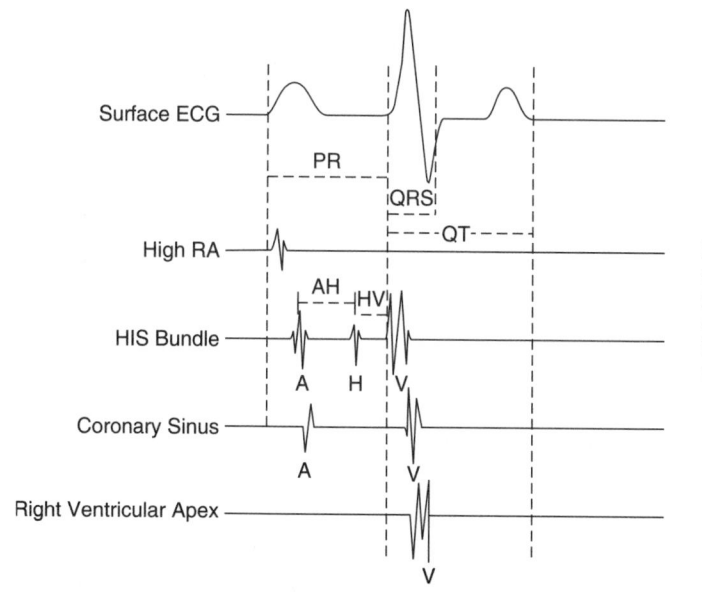

**Figure 2-7** • Measurement of surface and intracardiac conduction intervals. The interrupted vertical lines represent calipers. Refer to Table 2–2 for a description of measurement reference points.

not affected by autonomic tone but is influenced by antiarrhythmic medications. Typical baseline intervals, points of measurement, and normal values are summarized in Table 2–2.

## Programmed Stimulation Protocols

Programmed stimulation is a technique that involves delivery of stimuli to the atrium or ventricle to evaluate the conduction system. Programmed stimulation protocols provide an opportunity to assess cardiac refractory periods, conduction properties, and automaticity. The presence and characteristics of reentrant circuits are also studied.

A refractory period is the interval after depolarization during which a cell cannot be depolarized again. The refractory period of cardiac tissue is characterized by the tissue's response to premature paced impulses. A delivered premature impulse fails to propagate through tissue that is refractory. The effective refractory period (ERP) of a tissue is the longest coupling interval for which a premature impulse fails to propagate through that tissue. Simply, it refers to the latest premature impulse delivered that is blocked; if the premature impulse were delivered any later, the recovered tissue would propagate the impulse. The effective refractory periods of the atria, AV node, and ventricle are assessed during the EP study. These parameters are summarized in Chart 2–4.

Other programmed stimulation protocols are detailed in subsequent chapters. The sinus node recovery time stimulation protocol is discussed in Chapter 4, and arrhythmia induction techniques are presented in Chapters 6, 7, and 8.

| **Table 2-2** ELECTROPHYSIOLOGY STUDY BASELINE INTERVALS | | |
|---|---|---|
| **INTERVAL** | **MEASUREMENT** | **NORMAL RANGE (MS)** |
| Surface ECG | | |
| PR interval | Onset of P wave to onset of QRS complex | 120–150 |
| QRS duration | Onset of QRS complex to end of QRS complex | 80–110 |
| QT interval | Onset of QRS complex to end of T wave | 250–400 |
| Corrected QT | Divide QT interval by the square root of R to R interval | Normal range corrected to heart rate |
| Intracardiac ECG | | |
| AH interval | Earliest rapid atrial deflection to onset of His deflection on His electrogram | 65–140 |
| HV interval | Earliest His deflection on His electrogram to earliest surface ECG ventricular activation | 33–55 |

## Chart 2-4
### PROTOCOLS USED TO EVALUATE EFFECTIVE REFRACTORY PERIODS

Atrial effective refractory period (AERP)
- Method: atrial pace (A1) with the introduction of premature stimuli (A2) using even shorter A1–A2 intervals until an atrial response cannot be elicited; the first A2 that does not capture (meaning it is blocked)
- AERP value is the longest coupling interval (S1–S2) that fails to capture
- Normal values: 150–360 ms
- Purpose: provide an indication of the atrium's ability to respond and maintain atrial arrhythmias Figure 2–8 depicts an atrial effective refractory period.

AV node effective refractory period (AVNERP)
- Method: atrial pace (A1) drive train × 8 impulses at cycle lengths between 400 and 600 ms with the introduction of premature stimuli (A2) using shorter (S1–S2) intervals until AV block occurs (*Note:* As the A2 is delivered closer to the A1, the AH interval is prolonged owing to the decremental conduction properties of the AV node.)
- AVNERP value is the longest premature cycle length where premature stimuli capture the atrium but fail to conduct through the AV node to the ventricles.
- Normal values: 230–450 ms

*continues*

### Chart 2-4
PROTOCOLS USED TO EVALUATE EFFECTIVE REFRACTORY PERIODS *(Continued)*

- Purpose: Assess AV node properties
  Figure 2–9 depicts an AV node effective refractory period.

Ventricular refractory period (VERP)

- Method: ventricular pace (V1) with the introduction of a premature stimuli (V2) using shortening coupling (V1–V2) intervals; as the premature stimuli (V2) are delivered closer to the ventricular drive train (V1), the ventricle fails to capture.
- VERP value is the longest (V1–V2) coupling interval that fails to capture the ventricle.
- Purpose: assess ventricular activation
  Figure 2–10 depicts a ventricular refractory period.

Decremental (decreasing cycle length) atrial and ventricular pacing protocol

- *Atrial method*: atrial (A1) pace at a rate slightly faster than the sinus rate and gradually increases the pacing rate until AV block (Wenckebach) occurs.
- Value may be referred to as atrial 1:1 conduction or as Wenckebach cycle length.
- Normal values: <540 ms
- Purpose: assess antegrade conduction properties

- *Ventricular method*: ventricular (V1) pace beginning at a rate slightly faster than the sinus rate and gradually increasing the pacing rate until VA block occurs (retrograde Wenckebach).
- Value is reported as the presence or absence of VA conduction
- Purpose: assess retrograde conduction
  Figure 2–11 depicts a decremental atrial pacing technique.

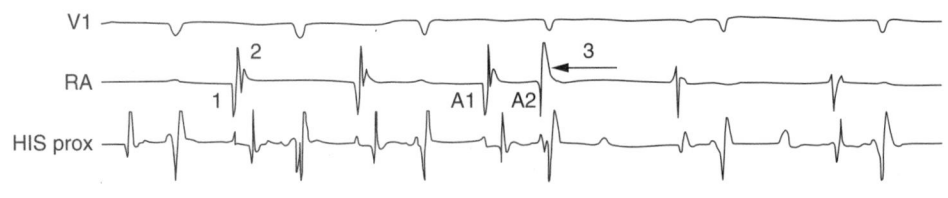

**Figure 2-8** • Electrogram depicts an atrial effective refractory period, which is the longest coupling interval (A1–A2) in which A2 fails to capture the atrium. In the RA tracing the first three complexes represent a pacing stimulus (1) followed by atrial depolarization (2). The fourth pacing stimulus, A2, defines the atrial effective refractory period because there is no capture of the atrium (3).

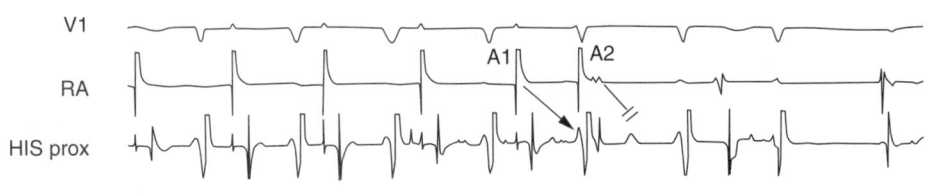

**Figure 2-9** • Electrogram depicts an AV node effective refractory period, which is the longest coupling interval (A1–A2) in which A2 captures the atrium but fails to conduct through the AV node. Arrow = conducts; oblique indicator ending in parallel horizontal lines = AV node block.

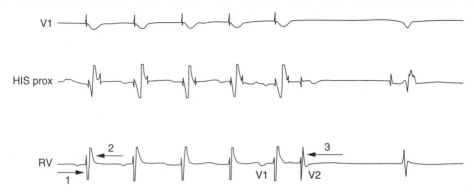

**Figure 2-10** • Electrogram depicts a ventricular refractory period which is the longest (V1–V2) coupling interval that falls to capture the ventricle. In the RV tracing the first five complexes represent a pacing stimulus (1) followed by ventricular depolarization (2). The sixth pacing stimulus, V2, defines the ventricular effective refractory period because there is no capture of the ventricle (3).

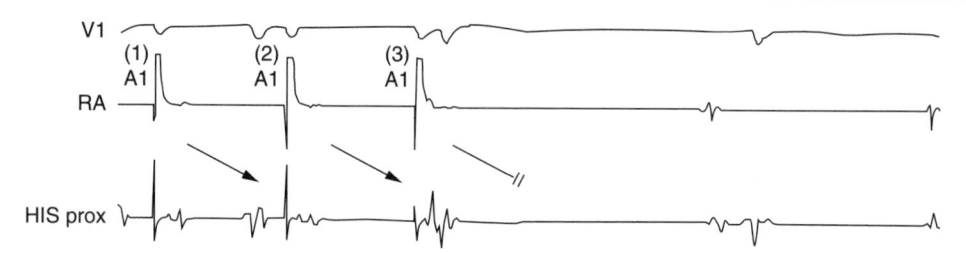

**Figure 2-11** • Electrograms depict a decremental atrial pacing protocol which is pacing at faster rates (or shorter cycle lengths) until AV block occurs. In the RA tracing, during atrial overdrive pacing the first two complexes (1) and (2) show the development of Wenckebach (and progressively longer PR intervals) until the third complex (3) does not conduct through the AV node (blocked).

## DEFIBRILLATION TECHNIQUES

Termination of induced ventricular arrhythmias is achieved by one of two methods: programmed stimulation or direct current (DC) cardioversion/defibrillation. Programmed stimulation to terminate ventricular tachycardia is attempted by pacing 8–12 beats at a cycle length 10–20 ms faster than the cycle length of the tachycardia. Pacing is repeated at faster rates if the original attempt is unsuccessful. Accelerating the tachycardia or causing it to degenerate to ventricular fibrillation is possible and usually requires rescue shock defibrillation.

Direct current cardioversion/defibrillation is immediately administered in the event the patient loses consciousness. The energy can be efficiently and safely delivered through "hands-free" defibrillation pads, shown in Figure 2–12, or defibrillation paddles.

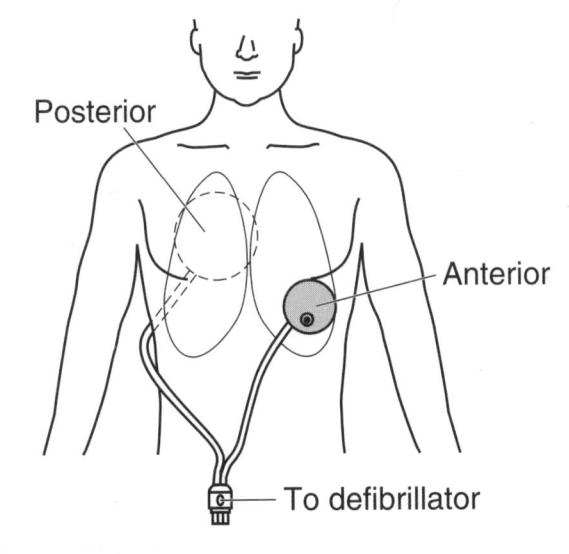

Posterior

Anterior

To defibrillator

**Figure 2–12** • Example of "hands-free" pacing/defibrillating pads. Location of the pad position may vary owing to the clinical application. This example shows one pad (electrode) placed on the anterior chest and the other on the back.

# CHAPTER 3

# CARE OF THE PATIENT UNDERGOING AN ELECTROPHYSIOLOGY STUDY

Care of the patient undergoing an electrophysiology (EP) study and ablation is similar to that of the patient undergoing cardiac catheterization. The three phases of care—preprocedure, intraprocedure, and postprocedure—are discussed in the following text.

## PREPROCEDURAL CARE

Care of the patient prior to an EP procedure focuses on determining if the procedure is appropriate, conducting preliminary diagnostic testing, and educating the patient and family regarding what to expect during the continuum of care, including what will be required of them. Patients potentially requiring an EP study and ablation may be evaluated in the hospital or the electrophysiologist's office depending on the severity of the arrhythmia. Patients with arrhythmias that are not life-threatening may be evaluated outside the hospital setting; generally their procedures are also performed on an outpatient basis. Patients with more serious arrhythmias may have to be admitted to the hospital during an acute or first episode and so have their first contact with the electrophysiologist at that time.

Preprocedural screening ensures that the patient is a candidate for the procedure. The diagnostic test needed depends on the suspected arrhythmia. If procedures are determined to be appropriate, baseline laboratory values and an electrocardiogram (ECG) are obtained. Informed consent is obtained by the physician following a discussion of the reason for the procedure, risks involved, use of sedation, and alternatives. Preprocedural teaching is initiated and involves both the patient and family. Chart 3–1 lists the subjects discussed when educating the patient about EP procedures.

## INTRAPROCEDURAL CARE

Care immediately prior to and during the EP study involves preparing the patient for the procedure (application of monitoring devices and sterile readiness of the access site) and evaluating the patient's response to the procedure itself and the sedation, if given. Each EP department has its own standard of patient care for its procedures. Chart 3–2 describes a general standard of care for patients during an EP procedure.

## SEDATION/ANALGESIA

Intravenous administration of sedation agents may be appropriate for the conscious patient during the EP study to decrease anxiety, prevent excessive movement, and promote amnesia. The intravenous route of ad-

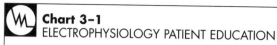

## Chart 3-1
### ELECTROPHYSIOLOGY PATIENT EDUCATION

- Explain the conduction system of the heart in terms understandable to the patient and family.
- Describe the purpose of an electrophysiology study.
- Discuss the known or suspected individual patient arrhythmia and the reason for the procedure.
- Discuss the need for a 12-lead electrogram.
- Discuss the need for baseline laboratory values including a negative pregnancy test in pre-menopausal or nonsterilized girls/women.
- Discuss weaning of current antiarrhythmic medications prior to the study.
- Provide written information or a video for the patient and the family.
- Discuss desire for preprocedural sedation.
- Instruct to withhold fluid and food beginning midnight prior to the procedure.
- Describe routine preparation for procedure: intravenous infusion, monitor, blood pressure cuff, pulse oximetry, and access site.
- Describe sensations the patient may experience during the procedure, such as local sedation for sheath insertion, rapid heart rates and skipped beats due to pacing, possibility of loss of consciousness, and effects of analgesics.

**Chart 3-2**
STANDARD OF CARE FOR ELECTROPHYSIOLOGY STUDIES

- Keep NPO for 6–12 hours.
- Have patient sign a consent form.
- Apply monitoring equipment: blood pressure (BP) cuff, ECG, pulse oximetry).
- Undertake sterile preparation and drape access site(s).
- Maintain patient intravenous infusion.
- Apply pace/defibrillate electrodes.

- Apply grounding pad to posterior scapula if having ablation.
- Monitor vital signs (blood pressure, pulse, respirations, oxygen saturation, level of consciousness, cardiac rhythm) at frequent intervals.
- Monitor patient response to analgesics or other medications.

ministration allows immediate absorption of the medication and titration of the dose specific to the patient's response. Formerly referred to as "conscious sedation," the 1996 American Society of Anesthesiologists Task Force has revised the term to "sedation/analgesia" to better define the objective of the sedative care provided. Sedation/analgesia refers to a reduced state of consciousness, the ability to tolerate unpleasant procedures, maintenance of adequate cardiopulmonary function, and the ability to respond to verbal commands or tactile stimulation.

Desirable effects of sedation include a slight initiation of slurred speech, cooperation, relaxation, diminished verbal communication, and easy arousal from sleep. Undesirable effects include agitation, combativeness, severely slurred speech, nonarousability from sleep, respiratory depression, hypotension, and apnea.

Prior to administration of sedation/analgesia, a qualified physician should evaluate and classify the patient's health status. A useful tool developed by the American Society of Anesthesiologists is shown in Table 3–1.

Each institution should develop their own protocol for administration of sedation/analgesia. Chart 3–3 outlines a general protocol for the care of the patient receiving intravenous sedation.

Medications used to induce sedation/analgesia generally fall into one of two categories: sedatives and narcotics. Table 3–2 describes the commonly used agents, usual dosage, administration guidelines, and adverse reactions. Information regarding reversal agents is contained in Table 3–3.

**Table 3–1** PHYSICAL STATUS CLASSIFICATION OF THE AMERICAN SOCIETY OF ANESTHESIOLOGISTS

| STATUS | DEFINITION |
|--------|------------|
| I | Normal, healthy patient |
| II | Patient with mild systemic disease |
| III | Patient with severe systemic disease that limits activity but is not incapacitating |
| IV | Patient with an incapacitating systemic disease |
| V | Moribund patient not expected to survive 24 hours with or without operation |

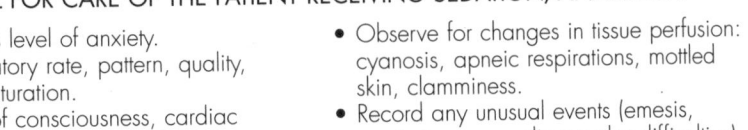

**Chart 3–3**
PROTOCOL FOR CARE OF THE PATIENT RECEIVING SEDATION/ANALGESIA

- Assess patient's level of anxiety.
- Monitor respiratory rate, pattern, quality, and oxygen saturation.
- Monitor level of consciousness, cardiac rhythm, blood pressure, and pulse at frequent intervals.
- Administer supplemental oxygen as needed.
- Have airway and suction equipment immediately available.

- Observe for changes in tissue perfusion: cyanosis, apneic respirations, mottled skin, clamminess.
- Record any unusual events (emesis, respiratory or cardiovascular difficulties).
- Document all medications, fluids administered, and blood and body fluids lost during the procedure.

## Table 3-2 SEDATIVE AND ANALGESIC AGENTS FOR ADULTS

| DRUG | USUAL DOSE | DOSING GUIDELINES | ADVERSE REACTIONS |
|---|---|---|---|
| Diazepam (Valium): benzodiazepine | Loading dose: 5–10 mg IVP slowly up to a total of 20 mg | Do not mix with other drugs<br>Give closely to IV cannula and inject slowly (5 mg/min)<br>Titrate to desired effect—slurred speech<br>Use with caution in elderly, chronically ill, decreased pulmonary reserve, ↓ kidney and/or hepatic function<br>Contraindicated in acute narrow-angle glaucoma<br>Reversal agent: Romazicon | Vein thrombosis, phlebitis, swelling and pain on IV injection (usually with small veins)<br>CV: bradycardia, cardiovascular collapse, hypotension<br>Increased respiratory depression when used with narcotics |
| Midazolam (Versed): benzodiazepine/ general anesthetic | <60 Years of age:<br>↑ 2.5 mg IVP over 2 min; wait 2 min to evaluate effect, then administer additional but not >5 mg total dose<br>With narcotics, ↓ dose by 30%<br>>60 Years of age: ↑ 1.5 mg | Caution with COPD or other high risk conditions, or receiving narcotics or other CNS depressants<br>Drug has been associated with respiratory depression and respiratory arrest when given IV<br>Use with caution in elderly, CHF, impaired renal or | Most common<br>Fluctuations in vital signs (↓ tidal volume, respiratory rate, apnea, variations in BP or heart rate)<br>Tenderness at IV site<br>Pain with injection<br>Hiccoughs<br>Nausea, vomiting |

| **Table 3-2** SEDATIVE AND ANALGESIC AGENTS FOR ADULTS *(Continued)* | | | |
|---|---|---|---|
| **DRUG** | **USUAL DOSE** | **DOSING GUIDELINES** | **ADVERSE REACTIONS** |
| | IVP over 2 min; wait 2 min to evaluate effect then administer additional but not >3.5 mg total dose With narcotics, ↓ dosing by 50% | excretory function Contraindicated in acute narrow-angle glaucoma if not being treated, acute ETOH intoxification, MAO inhibitors within 14 days Maintenance: 25% of dose used to first reach sedation endpoint Reversal agent: Romazicon 10 μg fentanyl = 1 mg morphine = 7.5 mg demerol Respiratory depressant effect may outlast sedative effect Reversal agent: Narcan | Less common Respiratory: laryngospasm, bronchospasm, wheezing CV: bigeminy, trigeminy PVCs, tachycardia, bradycardia CNS: confusion, argumentative-ness, retrograde amnesia |
| Fentanyl (Sublimaze): opiate agonist | Titrate dose to effect using 5–10 μg over 1–2 min | | Expect blurred vision and dry mouth Pain, burning on injection Respiratory depression, apnea, muscle rigidity including respiratory muscles, bradycardia, respiratory arrest, hyper/hypotension Do not administer if had MAO inhibitors within last 14 days Hypotension when used in conjection with Inapsine Agitation |

| | | | |
|---|---|---|---|
| Meperidine (Demerol): opiate agonist | 2–10 mg IVP/70 kg body weight | CI with MAO inhibitors within last 14 days<br>Titrate slowly<br>Reversal agent: Narcan | Respiratory depression, shock, cardiac arrest, lightheadedness, dizziness, nausea/vomiting, tachycardia, bradycardia |
| Nalbuphine (Nubain): partial opiate agonist | 10 mg IVP/70 kg body weight; repeat 3–6 hr | Use with caution in hepatic- or renal-impaired patients<br>Reversal agent: Romazicon | Respiratory and circulatory depression<br>Clamminess, nausea/vomiting, vertigo, dry mouth<br>Patients who are narcotic-dependent may experience withdrawal symptoms with this drug |
| Morphine: opiate agonist | Not typically used for conscious sedation<br>2–10 mg IVP/70 kg body weight over 4–5 min | Reduced dose for elderly or for renal or hepatic failure<br>Reversal agent: Narcan | Urticaria<br>Hypotension<br>Bronchoconstriction<br>Respiratory depression<br>High doses cause excitement, convulsions, nausea/vomiting |

COPD = chronic obstructive pulmonary disease; CNS = central nervous system; CHF = chronic heart failure; ETOH = ethyl alcohol; MAO = monoamine oxidase; CV = cardiovascular; BP = blood pressure; PVCs = premature ventricular contractions; CI = cardiac insufficiency.

| Table 3–3 | SEDATIVE AND ANALGESIC AGENTS FOR ADULTS | | |
| --- | --- | --- | --- |
| **AGENT** | **USUAL DOSE** | **DOSING GUIDELINES** | **ADVERSE REACTIONS** |
| Naloxone (Narcan) | Partial reversal: 0.1–0.2 mg slow IVP at 2 to 3 min intervals until effect<br>Full reversal: 0.4 mg IVP | IV doses last only 20–30 min; narcotic may outlast effects of reversal agents<br>Caution with preexisting heart disease | Pulmonary edema<br>Excitation<br>Hypotension, tachycardia<br>Ventricular tachycardia<br>Ventricular fibrillation<br>Seizure activity in habitual narcotic users |
| Flumazenil (Romazicon) | Initial dose of 2.5 mg IVP over 15 sec; after 45 sec repeat 0.2 mg<br>Repeat 0.2 mg/min up to 1 mg | Administer no >3 mg/hr<br>Monitor for resedation | Risk of seizure when given in the presence of long-term benzodiazepine use and cyclic antidepressant overdose |

Discontinuation of a sedation/analgesia protocol may be accomplished by meeting previously established discontinuation criteria. Chart 3–4 provides general criteria on which to base discontinuation of a sedation/analgesia regimen.

## POSTPROCEDURAL CARE

Postprocedural care of the patient who has undergone an EP procedure includes assessment of hemodynamic status and the development of complications, such as bleeding from access sites, cardiac tamponade, or distal thrombosis. A general standard of care for the patient recovering from an EP procedure is described in Chart 3–5.

Discharge instructions are provided to the patient and family after the bed rest period is complete. These instructions are summarized in Chart 3–6.

### Chart 3-4
### CRITERIA FOR DISCONTINUATION OF A SEDATION/ANALGESIA REGIMEN

- Stable vital signs and oxygen saturation
- Return of presedation level of consciousness; patient is completely arousable and responsive or responds appropriately for age; or both
- Able to ambulate with minimal assistance if tolerated by physical status and procedure

### Chart 3-5
### GENERAL STANDARD OF CARE AFTER ELECTROPHYSIOLOGY STUDY

- Maintain bed rest with head of bed no more than 30 degrees; keep affected leg straight for 2–3 hours for venous access and 6 hours for arterial access.
- Medicate for back discomfort related to bed rest.
- Monitor vital signs at frequent intervals (blood pressure, heart rate, respiratory rate, oxygen saturation).
- Monitor access site for bleeding or hematoma.
- Monitor pulses distal to the access site.

**Chart 3-6**
DISCHARGE INSTRUCTIONS FOR THE ELECTROPHYSIOLOGY STUDY PATIENT

- Encourage ambulation for 24 hours.
- Clarify medications including discontinuation of antiarrhythmic drugs if appropriate.
- Instruct patient regarding the signs and symptoms of bleeding at the access site and what measures to take.
- Instruct the patient regarding the signs and symptoms of infection and what measures to take.
- Provide information regarding when to follow up with the physician.
- Instruct patient not to drive or engage in potentially high risk activities for 12 hours after receiving sedation agents.

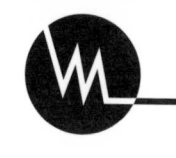

The sinus node is a crescent-shaped structure that lies just underneath the epicardium at the junction of the superior vena cava and the right atrium (Figure 4–1). It is composed of cells that have the feature of automaticity (the ability to depolarize spontaneously). The sinus node is the site from which a normal sinus P wave is generated. The sinus node region is richly innervated by fibers from both the sympathetic and parasympathetic arms of the autonomic nervous system.

## CLINICAL MANIFESTATIONS OF DYSFUNCTION

Sick sinus syndrome is the most common clinical condition involving the sinus node. It usually manifests as:

1. Persistent sinus bradycardia
2. Chronotropic incompetence (inappropriately low heart rate response during exercise)
3. Intermittent sinus pauses
4. Paroxysms of atrial fibrillation with pauses upon termination of the fibrillation

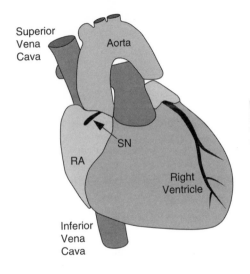

**Figure 4–1** • Typical position of the sinus node (SN). It is located at the junction of the superior vena cava and the anterior right atrium (RA) and extends inferiorly along the lateral aspect of the right atrial wall.

Presenting symptoms are most often syncope, presyncope, or exercise intolerance. There may be associated palpitations in patients with atrial tachyarrhythmias. Patient with sinus node dysfunction are often highly sensitive to cardiac medications, such as calcium channel blockers, β-blockers, and antiarrhythmic agents. These medications must be used with caution as they tend to worsen the bradyarrhythmias and may induce periods of asystole.

## ETIOLOGY OF DYSFUNCTION

Sinus node dysfunction may be due to extrinsic or intrinsic causes. The most common extrinsic causes of abnormal sinus node function are enhanced vagal tone (i.e., carotid sinus hypersensitivity) and administration of pharmacologic agents (Table 4–1). Intrinsic sinus node dysfunction is due to an abnormality in the function of the sinus node cells themselves: in those that generate the impulse or those that conduct the impulse to the atrium. In patients with intrinsic sinus node dysfunction, an increased amount of fibrosis is often found in and around the sinus node.

| **Table 4–1** | MEDICATIONS THAT COMMONLY DEPRESS SINUS NODE FUNCTION |
|---|---|
| β-Blockers | Antiarrhythmic agents |
| Calcium channel blockers | Digitalis |
| Sympatholytic agents | |

# EVALUATION OF SINUS NODE FUNCTION

The most frequently used measures of sinus node function in the electrophysiology (EP) laboratory are the sinus node recovery time (SNRT) and the corrected sinus node recovery time (CSNRT). Other measurements that may be helpful are the sinoatrial conduction time and the sinus node refractory period, although these measurements are more cumbersome and are of doubtful clinical significance.

The sinus node recovery time is measured by pacing the right atrium at various cycle lengths, abruptly terminating the pacing and measuring the interval from the last paced beat to the first sinus recovery beat (Figure 4–2). A fairly standard protocol for measuring the SNRT is to use pacing cycle lengths of 600, 500, 400, 350, and 300 ms and pace for 30–60 seconds. The normal maximum sinus node recovery time is 1.5 seconds or less. The CSNRT is calculated by subtracting the baseline sinus cycle length (SCL) from the SNRT (CSNRT = SNRT – SCL); its normal value is 550 ms or less. The sensitivity of the SNRT and CSNRT for detecting abnormal sinus node function is approximately 70%.

## CLINICAL UTILITY

Measuring sinus node function in the EP laboratory is used mainly to determine if sinus node dysfunction is a potential cause of syncope of unknown etiology. In general, patients with no other explanation for their syncope who have prolonged SNRTs benefit from pacemaker placement. This is especially true in patients with markedly prolonged SNRTs (i.e., > 2.5 seconds). Patients with abnormal sinus node function who are given agents with sinus node depressant properties (Table 4–1) must be observed carefully, often with in-hospital monitoring or follow-up Holter monitoring to minimize the risk of serious bradyarrhythmias.

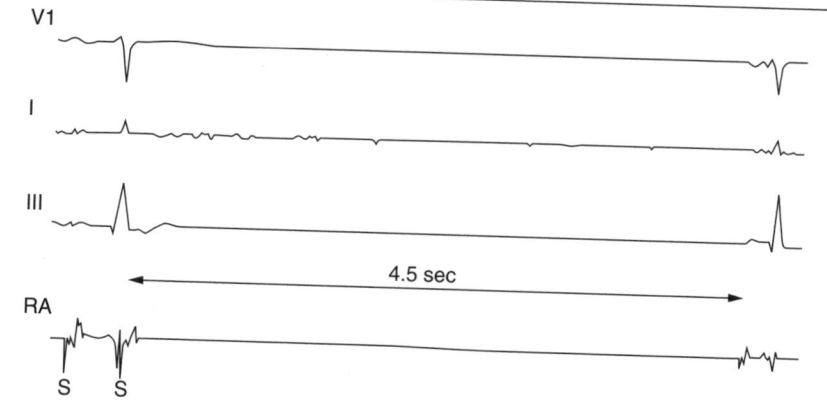

**Figure 4–2 •** Sinus node recovery time (SNRT) is determined by pacing the right atrium (RA) at rapid rates, abruptly terminating pacing, and then measuring the time from the last paced beat to the first spontaneous atrial beat. Shown are recordings from surface leads $V_1$, I, and III and intracardiac recordings from the right atrium (RA). The atrium was paced (S) at a cycle length of 350 ms for 30 seconds, and then pacing was stopped. The measured SNRT was 4.5 seconds (normal SNRT ≤ 1.5 seconds).

# ATRIOVENTRICULAR CONDUCTION

Normal atrioventricular (AV) conduction has two components: conduction through the AV node and conduction through the His-Purkinje system. It is usually the AV node that limits conduction to the ventricles. The AV node and the origin of the His bundle are located at the junction of the atrial septum and the summit of the ventricular septum. The electrical activity of this region may be recorded by placing a catheter across the superomedial portion of the tricuspid annulus (Figure 5–1).

The AV node, like the sinus node, is richly innervated by the parasympathetic and sympathetic limbs of the autonomic nervous system. An increase in vagal tone decreases AV node conduction, whereas enhanced sympathetic tone improves AV node conduction. The effects of the autonomic nervous system on His-Purkinje conduction are minimal and usually not of clinical importance.

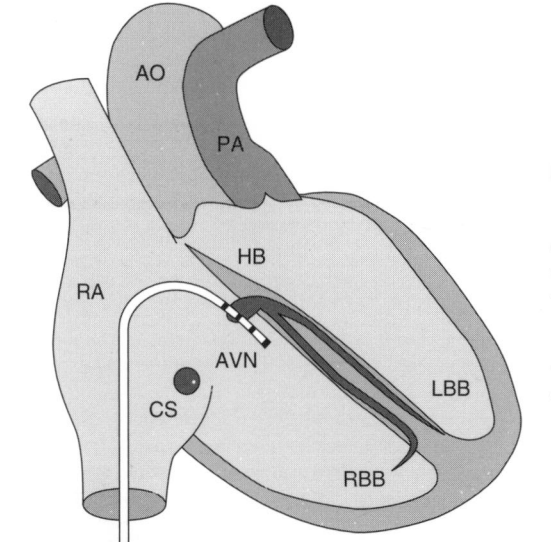

**Figure 5-1 •** Location of the AV node (AVN), His bundle (HB), and right (RBB) and left (LBB) bundle branches. The His bundle recording catheter is positioned along the tricuspid annulus at its superomedial aspect to record the His bundle electrogram. This position allows simultaneous recording of low right atrial electrical activity, the His bundle electrogram, and the right ventricular electrogram. RA: right atrium; CS: coronary sinus; AO: aorta; PA: pulmonary artery.

## EVALUATING AV NODE FUNCTION

The three primary measures of AV node function are the AH interval, AV block cycle length (AVBCL), and AV node effective refractory period (AVNERP). The AH interval is a measure of the conduction time through the AV node and is measured between the atrial electrogram and the His bundle electrogram on the His bundle recording catheter (Figure 5–2). The AVBCL is the longest pacing cycle length at which conduction through the AV junction is blocked. In most patients this block occurs at the AV node level, so one sees an atrial electrogram without a corresponding His bundle or ventricular electrogram with the blocked beat. When the block occurs in the AV node, the AVBCL is also known as the Wenckebach block cycle length, as there is a progressive increase in the AH (and PR) interval just prior to the blocked beat as with Wenckebach type block (Figure 5–3).

The AVNERP is measured using the extrastimulus pacing technique. A drive train of usually eight impulses (A1) is delivered in the high right atrium, and an extrastimulus (A2) is delivered at the end of the drive train at progressively shorter coupling intervals until the impulse blocks in the AV node. The AVNERP is defined as the longest atrial coupling interval (A1–A2) that blocks in the AV node (Figure 5–4). The AVNERP is commonly measured using drive train cycle lengths (A1–A1) of 400–600 ms. Typical values for normal AV node function are shown in Table 5–1.

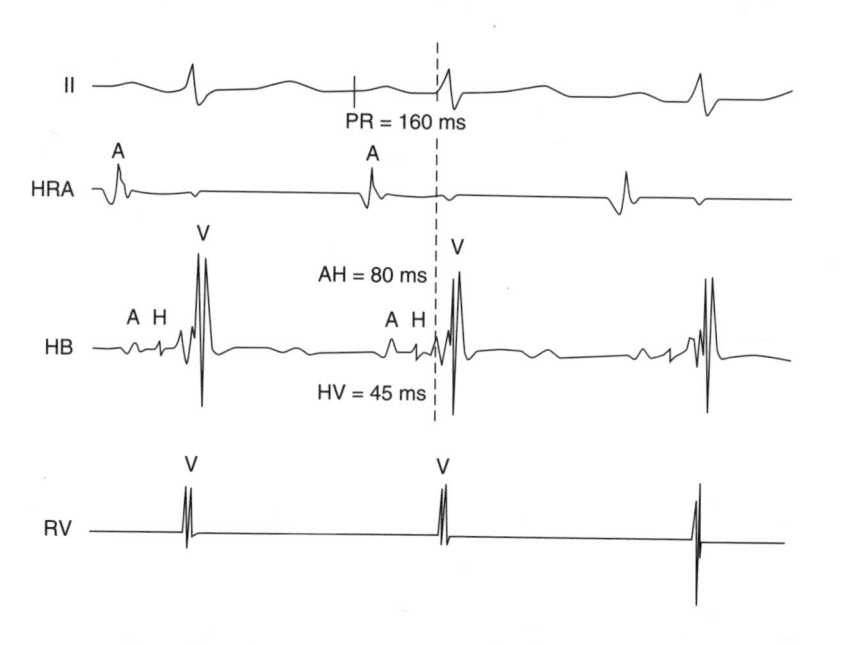

**Figure 5-2** • Typical electrogram recordings from a patient during normal sinus rhythm and with normal AV conduction. The electrode catheters are positioned in the high right atrium (HRA), His bundle recording position (HB), and right ventricle (RV), which are standard recording locations. The PR interval, which is a reflection of conduction through the atrium and AV junction, is measured from the onset of the P wave to the onset of the QRS complex using one of the standard surface ECG leads. In this case, the PR interval measured 160 ms in lead II. The AH interval is measured between the atrial electrogram (A) and the His bundle electrogram (H) on the His bundle recording catheter (HB). The AH interval determines the conduction time through the AV node and in this case measured 80 ms. The HV interval is measured between the His bundle electrogram (H) and the onset of the surface QRS complex. The HV interval measures the conduction time through the infranodal conduction system (His bundle, bundle branches, and Purkinje fibers). In this recording, the HV interval measured 45 ms.

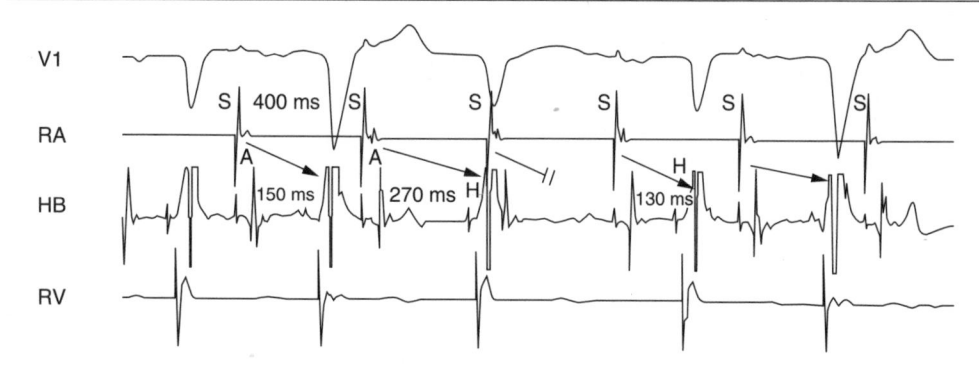

**Figure 5-3 •** Typical AV node Wenckebach behavior during atrial overdrive pacing. Recordings are made from surface lead $V_1$, and intracardiac recordings are from the right atrium (RA), His bundle region (HB), and right ventricle (RV). Atrial overdrive pacing was performed at a cycle length (S–S) of 400 ms. Note that there is progressive PR and AH prolongation just prior to the blocked beat and shortening of the AH interval after the blocked beat.

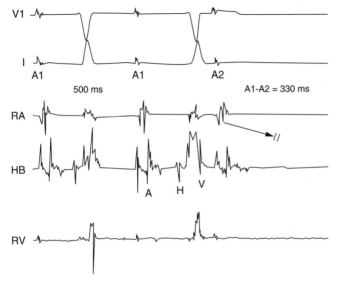

**Figure 5-4** • Measurement of the AV node effective refractory period (AVNERP). Shown are recordings from surface leads $V_1$ and I and intracardiac recordings from the right atrium (RA), His bundle region (HB), and right ventricle (RV). The AVNERP is determined by pacing the right atrium at a specific cycle length (A1–A1) using a drive train of eight impulses and delivering a premature beat at progressively shorter coupling intervals (A1–A2). Here only the last two paced beats of the drive train A1–A1 = 500 ms are shown; the A1–A2 coupling interval is 330 ms. The A2 paced beat blocked in the AV node. This was the longest A1–A2 coupling interval that blocked in the AV node, and therefore the AVNERP was 330 ms.

| Table 5-1 | TYPICAL VALUES FOR NORMAL AV NODE FUNCTION |
|-----------|---------------------------------------------|
| **MEASUREMENT** | **VALUE (ms)** |
| AH interval | 65-140 |
| AVBCL | 350-450 |
| AVNERP* | 220-320 |

AH: atrial-His bundle; AVBCL: atrioventricular block cycle length; AVNERP: atrioventricular node effective refractory period.
 *Measured using a drive train cycle length of 500 ms.

## HIS-PURKINJE SYSTEM CONDUCTION

Infranodal (His-Purkinje) conduction is first evaluated by measuring the HV interval (Figure 5-2). This interval is the time it takes an impulse to travel through the His bundle, bundle branches, and Purkinje fibers to the ventricles. The HV interval should be measured from the His bundle deflection to the start of the surface QRS complex. The normal duration of the HV interval is 35-55 ms. Table 5-2 notes various HV interval measurements and their clinical significance. A value of less than 35 ms for the HV interval indicates ventricular preexcitation (Wolff-Parkinson-White syndrome) may be present if the recording catheter is advanced too far into the right ventricle and is actually recording the right bundle branch electrogram

**Table 5-2** HV INTERVAL MEASUREMENTS AND THEIR CLINICAL IMPLICATIONS

| MEASURED HV INTERVAL (ms) | COMMENT |
| --- | --- |
| 35–55 | Normal |
| <35 | Ventricular preexcitation, possible right bundle branch recording |
| 55–70 | Mild prolongation of little clinical significance, common with left bundle branch block |
| 70–100 | Moderate prolongation; permanent pacemaker may be indicated in patients with syncope of unknown etiology |
| >100 | Severe prolongation; high risk for complete AV block; permanent pacing indicated |

(Figure 5–5). To ensure that a true His bundle deflection is being measured, the catheter must be placed proximal enough such that a good-sized atrial electrogram, His bundle deflection and ventricular electrogram are recorded. If a proper recording is made and the HV interval measured is still less than 35 ms, it is indicative of an accessory AV connection that bypasses the normal AV conduction system and preexcites the ventricle. In patients with ventricular preexcitation, the HV interval tends to shorten with atrial overdrive pacing because the accessory pathway conduction time remains relatively fixed at different pacing rates, whereas the AV nodal conduction time (AH interval) increases with faster pacing rates.

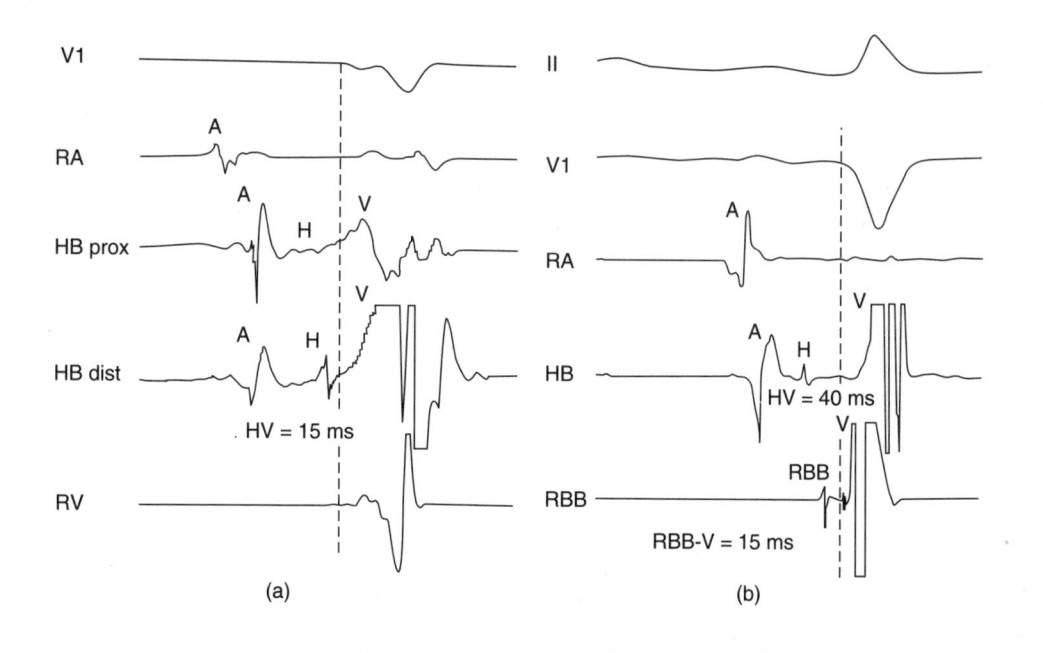

| V1 | | II | |
|---|---|---|---|
| RA | A | V1 | |
| HB prox | A  H  V | RA | A |
| HB dist | A  H  V | HB | A  H  V |
| | HV = 15 ms | | HV = 40 ms |
| RV | | RBB | V  RBB |
| | | | RBB-V = 15 ms |
| (a) | | (b) | |

**Figure 5-5 • (a)** Ventricular preexcitation. These recordings, from a patient with Wolff-Parkinson-White (WPW) syndrome, demonstrate overt ventricular preexcitation. Shown are a recording from surface lead $V_1$ and intra-cardiac recordings from the right atrium (RA), proximal His bundle region (HB prox), distal His bundle region (HB dist), and right ventricle (RV). The His bundle distal recording showed a sizable atrial (A), His bundle (H), and ventricular (V) electrogram. The HV interval, measured from the His bundle electrogram (H) to the onset of the surface QRS complex, is 15 ms, indicating the presence of ventricular preexcitation. **(b)** Normal AV conduction. These recordings, from a patient with normal AV conduction, show recordings from surface leads II and $V_1$ and intra-cardiac recordings from the right atrium (RA), His bundle region (HB), and right bundle branch region (RBB). The HV interval is normal, measuring 40 ms. The RBB-V interval is also within normal limits and measured 15 ms. One can see that if the His bundle catheter was mistakenly placed more distally in the RBB region and the RBB electrogram was mistaken for the His bundle electrogram, it could lead to the erroneous diagnosis of ventricular preexcitation (see text). To avoid this problem, it is important to make sure that the His bundle catheter records a sizable atrial electrogram as well as a His bundle and ventricle electrogram when the HV interval is measured.

A prolonged HV interval indicates that there is disease in the His-Purkinje system that is delaying conduction to the ventricle. Mild degrees of HV prolongation (55–70 ms) are usually of little clinical significance. Marked HV prolongation (>100 ms) (Figure 5–6) and episodes of infra-His block (Figure 5–7) are generally considered indications for permanent pacemaker placement. These patients have an approximately 25% chance of developing complete heart block over a 1-year period. In patients with symptoms of syncope or presyncope and moderate degrees of HV prolongation (70–100 ms), the possibility of intermittent high grade infra-His block must be considered. Pacemaker placement should be considered in these patients, although documentation of a greater degree of infranodal block should be attempted. Atrial overdrive pacing down to a cycle length of at least 400 ms should be attempted to induce infranodal block. If AV nodal block limits conduction to the His-Purkinje system at pacing cycle lengths of more than 400 ms, atropine or isoproterenol can be given to improve AV nodal function and allow 1:1 conduction to the His bundle. This maneuver is important because when block occurs in the AV node the His-Purkinje system cannot be adequately evaluated.

Another technique for stressing the His-Purkinje system is to administer intravenous procainamide. Class 1A antiarrhythmics such as procainamide impair conduction through the His bundle. Patients who develop significant HV prolongation (>100 ms) or infranodal block after intravenous procainamide should be considered for pacemaker placement, especially if a class I antiarrhythmic agent is to be utilized or if the patient has syncope of unknown etiology.

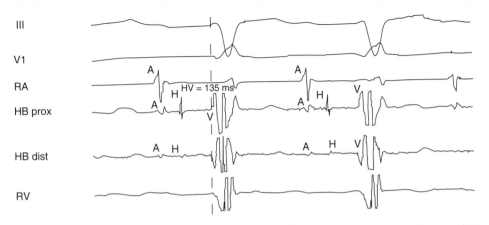

**Figure 5–6** • These recordings are from a patient with severe infranodal conduction system disease and HV prolongation. The recordings are from surface leads III and V₁ and intracardiac recordings from the right atrium (RA), proximal (HB prox) and distal (HB distal) His bundle regions, and the right ventricle (RV). The HV interval measured 135 ms, indicating the presence of severe infranodal conduction system disease and a high risk for progression to complete heart block. In general, an HV interval of more than 100 ms is an indication for pacemaker implantation.

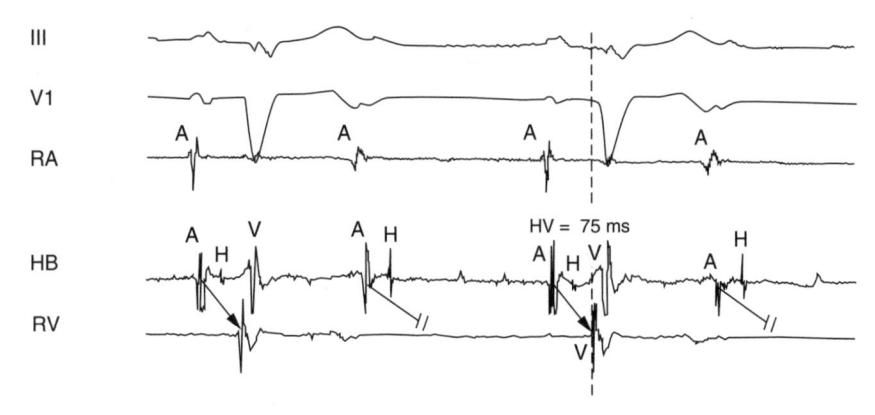

**Figure 5-7 •** These recordings are from a patient with a history of aortic stenosis and recurrent syncope. Shown are recordings from surface leads III and $V_1$ and intracardiac recordings from the right atrium (RA), His bundle region (HB), and right ventricle (RV). The baseline HV interval measured 75 ms. The patient developed spontaneous 2:1 AV block below the His bundle, indicating the need for pacemaker implantation.

# CHAPTER 6

# PAROXYSMAL SUPRAVENTRICULAR TACHYCARDIA

Paroxysmal supraventricular tachycardia (PSVT) can be classified into three major types: (1) atrioventricular (AV) node reentrant tachycardia; (2) AV reentrant tachycardia; and (3) atrial tachycardia (Figure 6–1). During an electrophysiology study, an accurate diagnosis of the mechanism of the PSVT can be made quickly using some simple criteria. The purpose of this chapter is to describe how to diagnose the most common forms of PSVT. An explanation of the differential diagnosis of more unusual and complex forms of supraventricular tachycardia can be found in standard electrophysiology texts.

## AV NODE REENTRANT TACHYCARDIA

Typical AV node reentrant tachycardia (AVNRT) is the most common form of PSVT in the adult population, accounting for up to 80% of cases. The atypical form of AVNRT is much less common than the typical form and is seen as the primary arrhythmia in fewer than 5% of PSVT cases. This section describes the characteristic electrophysiologic features of typical AV node reentrant tachycardia.

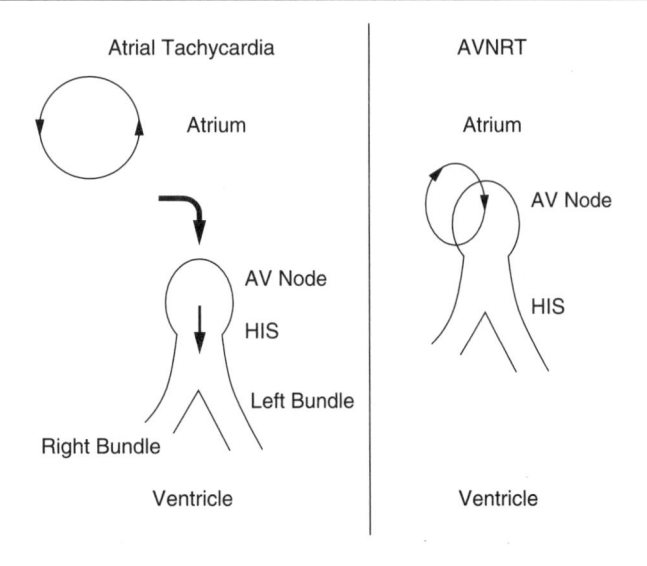

AVRT

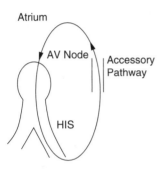

Atrium

AV Node

Accessory
Pathway

HIS

Ventricle

**Figure 6-1 •** Three types of paroxysmal supraventricular tachycardia (PSVT). With atrial tachycardia, the arrhythmia circuit or focus is localized entirely in the atrium. The reentrant circuit for AV node reentrant tachycardia (AVNRT) is thought to involve the AV node and adjacent perinodal atrial tissue. In atrioventricular reentrant tachycardia (AVRT), which utilizes an accessory pathway, the circuit includes the atrium, AV node, His-Purkinje system, ventricle, and accessory pathway.

## Pathophysiology

AVNRT is a reentrant arrhythmia whose circuit is confined to an area within or in close proximity to the AV node (Figure 6–1). This circuit probably involves both AV nodal and perinodal atrial tissue. In patients with AVNRT there are at least two AV nodal pathways. In the typical form there are both fast and slow AV nodal pathways. During tachycardia the slow pathway conducts antegrade to the ventricle, and the fast pathway conducts retrograde to the atrium. The presence of dual AV nodal physiology (i.e., the presence of both fast and slow pathways) is usually determined using atrial extrastimulus pacing techniques. Extrastimuli are delivered at progressively shorter coupling intervals, and the AH interval is measured. An increase in the AH interval of 50 ms or more, corresponding to shortening of the extrastimulus coupling interval by 10 ms, is defined as an AV nodal "jump" and indicates the presence of dual AV nodal pathways (Figure 6–2).

## Induction and Diagnosis

Typical AVNRT is usually induced using atrial overdrive pacing or atrial extrastimulation. During normal sinus rhythm the impulse usually travels antegrade through the AV node via the fast pathway. Because the fast pathway typically has a longer block cycle length and longer refractory period than the slow pathway, rapid atrial pacing and short coupled atrial extrastimuli often cause block in the fast pathway with conduction down the slow pathway. This then allows retrograde conduction to occur up the fast pathway with

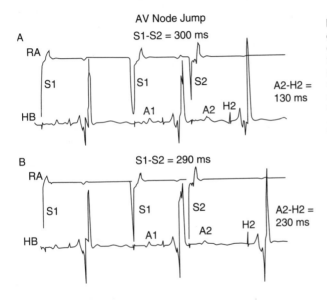

AV Node Jump

**A**

RA

S1

S1-S2 = 300 ms

S1    S2

A2-H2 = 130 ms

HB    A1    A2  H2

**B**

RA

S1-S2 = 290 ms

S1    S2

A2-H2 = 230 ms

HB    A1    A2  H2

**Figure 6-2** • AV nodal jump. Intracardiac recordings from the right atrium (RA) and His bundle region (HB). Pacing of the right atrium was performed using an eight-beat drive train (S1–S1 = 500 ms), of which only the last two beats are shown, and a premature stimulus (S2) was delivered at progressively shorter intervals. **(A)** S1–S2 coupling interval was 300 ms with a corresponding A2–H2 interval of 130 ms. **(B)** S1–S2 coupling interval was decreased by 10 ms to 290 ms, and the A2–H2 interval increased to 230 ms. The increase of the A2–H2 interval by ≥50 ms with a decrease of the S1–S2 coupling interval by 10 ms defines the presence of an AV nodal jump and indicates that dual AV nodal physiology is present. A = atrial electrogram; H = His bundle electrogram; V = ventricular electrogram; S = pacing stimulus electrogram.

tachycardia induction (Figure 6–3). In some patients only a single retrograde atrial beat is seen after the impulse "jumps" onto the slow pathway. This is known as an AV nodal echo beat (Figure 6–4), and indicates that a potential AV node reentrant circuit is present. These patients may require the addition of atropine or isoproterenol to improve AV nodal conduction and allow for tachycardia induction.

In patients with AVNRT, the AV node must be able to conduct in the retrograde direction as well as the antegrade direction for there to be a complete circuit. Therefore when patients are being evaluated, ventricular pacing should be performed to detect ventriculoatrial (VA) conduction. In patients with typical AVNRT, retrograde conduction is via the fast pathway and the VA time is generally short. VA conduction is present in the baseline state in most patients, although some patients require the addition of isoproterenol or atropine to enhance AV nodal function and allow VA conduction to occur. Complete lack of VA conduction after the addition of AV nodal enhancing agents generally rules out AVNRT as the cause of a patient's tachycardia.

Electrophysiologic features characteristic of sustained typical AV node reentrant tachycardia are a short VA time with the earliest site of atrial activation recorded at the His bundle recording catheter ("concentric activation") (Figure 6–5). The VA time is usually 60 ms or less measured at the His bundle electrogram and 90 ms or less measured at the high right atrial electrogram.

Atrial and ventricular pacing maneuvers during tachycardia can also help identify the tachycardia type. One of the most useful maneuvers is ventricular overdrive pacing at cycle lengths that are less than the tachycardia cycle length. In patients with AVNRT ventricular overdrive pacing at rates greater than the tachycardia rate usually result in entrainment of the tachycardia. Entrainment is said to be present when the pacing results in acceleration of the tachycardia to the pacing rate and upon termination of pacing the tachycardia continues at its original rate and VA timing relationships (Figure 6–6). This finding is characteristic of supraventricular tachycardias that require VA conduction (e.g., AVNRT and accessory pathway tachycardia) but not atrial tachycardias. When entrainment with ventricular overdrive pacing is found, an atrial tachycardia can essentially be ruled out. The characteristic features of typical AV node reentrant tachycardia are summarized in Table 6–1.

## ACCESSORY PATHWAY TACHYCARDIAS

The second most common type of PSVT is orthodromic reciprocating tachycardia (ORT), which has an accessory pathway as one limb of its reentrant circuit (Figure 6–1). During ORT the impulse travels antegrade down the AV node to the ventricle and retrograde up the accessory pathway to the atrium. The purpose of this section is to describe how to diagnose the presence of an accessory pathway and evaluate for ORT. A description of other less common accessory pathway-mediated tachycardias can be found in more comprehensive electrophysiology texts.

### Accessory Pathway Types

Accessory pathways are muscle bundles that span the AV groove and connect the atrium and ventricle. They can be located almost anywhere along the tricuspid or mitral annulus but most commonly are located on the left side of the heart along the mitral annulus.

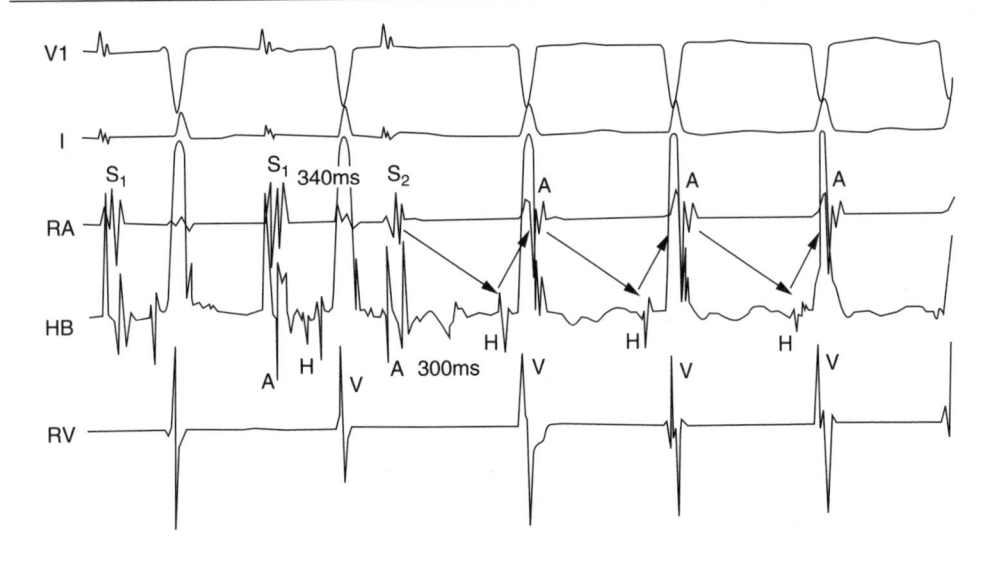

**Figure 6–3** • Induction of typical AV node reentrant tachycardia (AVNRT). Shown are recordings from surface leads V$_1$ and I and intracardiac recordings from the right atrium (RA), His bundle region (HB), and right ventricle (RV). AVNRT was induced by pacing the right atrium using an eight-beat drive train (S1–S1 = 500 ms), of which only the last two beats are shown, and delivering a premature extrastimulus (S2) with a coupling interval of 340 ms. At this S1–S2 coupling interval the antegrade conduction through the AV node was via the slow pathway (AH = 300 ms), conduction to the atrium returned via the fast pathway, and tachycardia was induced. Note that the ventricular electrogram (V) and the atrial electrogram (A) occur nearly simultaneously, which is characteristic of typical AVNRT. H = His bundle electrogram.

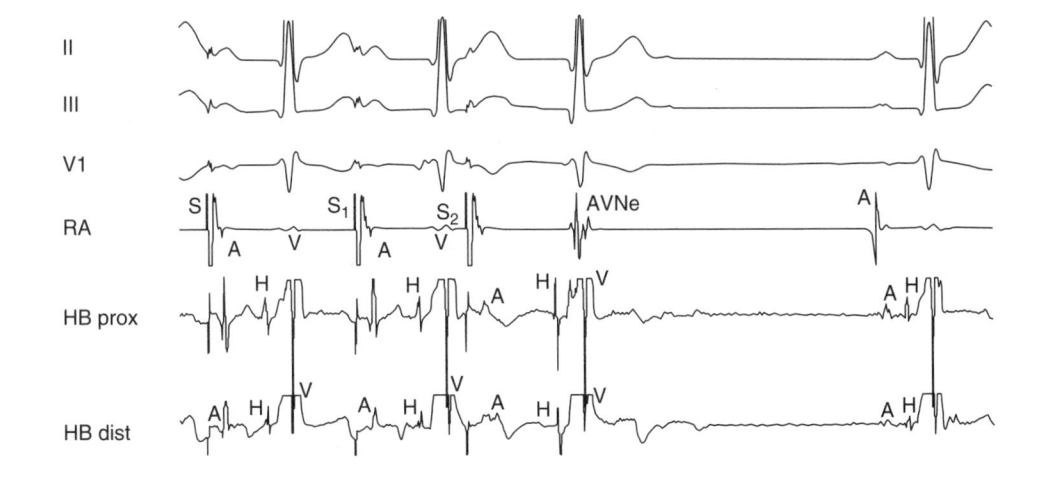

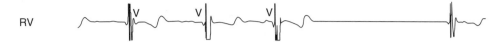

RV

**Figure 6–4** • AV node echo. Shown are recordings from surface leads II, III, and V₁ and intracardiac recordings from the right atrium (RA), proximal and distal His bundle region (HB prox, HB dist), and right ventricle (RV). The RA was paced using an eight-beat drive train (S1–S1 = 500 ms), of which only the last two are shown, and a premature stimulus (S2) was delivered at a coupling interval (S1–S2) of 350 ms. With this pacing scheme, a single AV nodal echo (AVNe) was seen. (See text). A, H, V = atrial, His bundle, and ventricular electrograms.

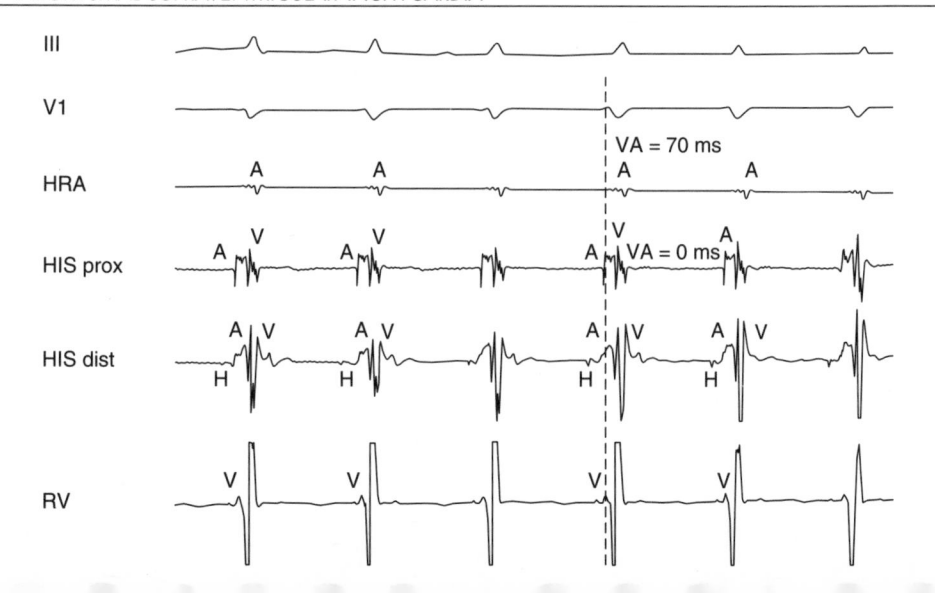

**Figure 6-5** • Earliest activation of the atrium at the His bundle recording region ("concentric activation") with a short ventriculoatrial (VA) activation time during typical AV nodal reentrant tachycardia (AVNRT). Shown are recordings from surface leads III and $V_1$ and intracardiac recordings from the high right atrium (HRA), proximal and distal His bundle region (HB prox, HB dist), and right ventricle (RV). The ventriculoatrial (VA) time during AVNRT is measured from the onset of the surface QRS to the local atrial electrocardiogram. The VA time was 0 ms at the His bundle region and 70 ms at the HRA. A VA time of ≤60 ms at the His bundle region and ≤90 ms at the HRA is indicative of typical AVRNT. A, H, V = atrial, His bundle, and ventricular electrograms.

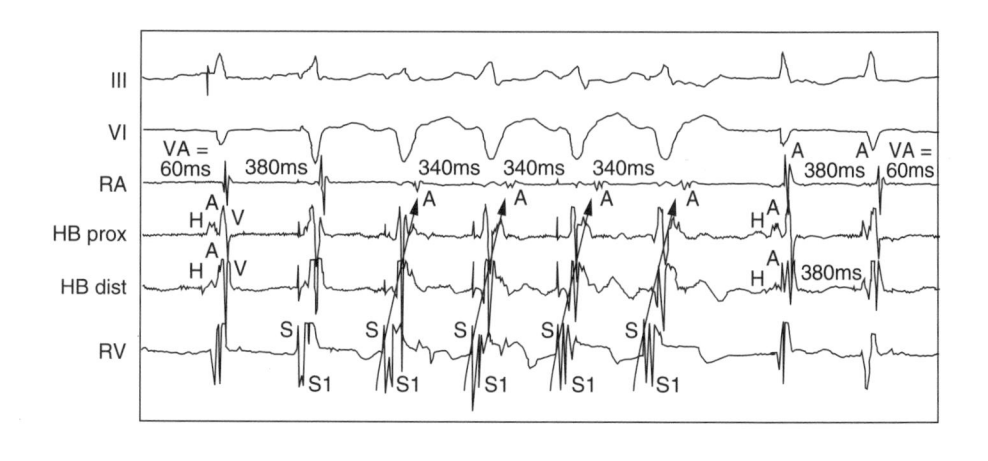

**Figure 6-6** • Entrainment of typical AV node reentrant tachycardia (AVNRT). These recordings are from a patient who was in typical AVNRT and underwent ventricular overdrive pacing for the purposes of entraining the tachycardia. Shown are recordings from surface leads III and $V_1$ and intracardiac recordings from the right atrium (RA), proximal and distal His bundle region (HB prox, HB dist), and right ventricle (RV). The tachycardia cycle length was 380 ms. Ventricular pacing (S) was performed at a cycle length of 340 ms. The last four beats of the five-beat drive train captured the ventricle and resulted in ventriculoatrial conduction and acceleration of the atrial rate to the pacing rate. Upon termination of pacing, the tachycardia resumed its previous rate and VA timing relationships. The timing relationship of the first postpacing tachycardia beat may be slightly altered because of the more rapid atrial rate during ventricular pacing. A, H, V, S = atrial, His bundle, ventricular, and pacing stimulus electrograms.

**Table 6-1** CHARACTERISTIC FEATURES OF PAROXYSMAL SUPRAVENTRICULAR TACHYCARDIAS

| FEATURE | TYPICAL AVNRT | ORT | ATRIAL TACHYCARDIA |
|---|---|---|---|
| VA timing at His bundle electrogram (ms) | ≤60 | >60; often >100 | Variable |
| Entrainment with ventricular pacing | Yes | Yes | No |
| Atrial activation | Concentric, earliest at His bundle position | Eccentric, earliest along the tricuspid or mitral annulus | Earliest at right or left atrial site; often "high to low" activation sequence |
| AV block with PSVT | Sometimes | Never | Common |

VA = ventriculoatrial; AVNRT = AV node reentrant tachycardia; ORT = orthodromic reciprocating tachycardia; PSVT = paroxysmal supraventricular tachycardia.

Overt accessory pathways are those that can conduct in the antegrade direction (from atrium to ventricle) and result in ventricular preexcitation, giving the characteristic ECG appearance of Wolff-Parkinson-White (WPW) syndrome (Figure 6–7) and shortening of the HV interval (<35 ms) (Figure 6–8). In most cases overt pathways can also conduct in the retrograde direction (from ventricle to atrium) and therefore may participate in ORTs. Concealed accessory pathways are those that conduct in only the retrograde direction. They cannot be detected on the surface ECG and do not result in shortening of the HV interval. Because they do conduct in the retrograde direction, they can participate in ORTs.

The characteristics of accessory pathway conduction are different from those of the AV node and are more like those of atrial or ventricular myocardium. The conduction time across an accessory pathway is usually short (<20 ms) compared to that of the AV node (AH intervals are usually >60 ms). These short conduction times can result in the atrial and ventricular electrograms seeming almost fused when recordings are made near the accessory pathway during pathway conduction (Figure 6–9). Unlike the AV node, conduction through an accessory pathway is nondecremental, which means that earlier extrastimuli and faster pacing rates do not result in progressive conduction delays through an accessory pathway as they do through the AV node. This difference between AV nodal and accessory pathway conduction, although sometimes helpful, is rarely the most important factor when diagnosing the presence of an accessory pathway.

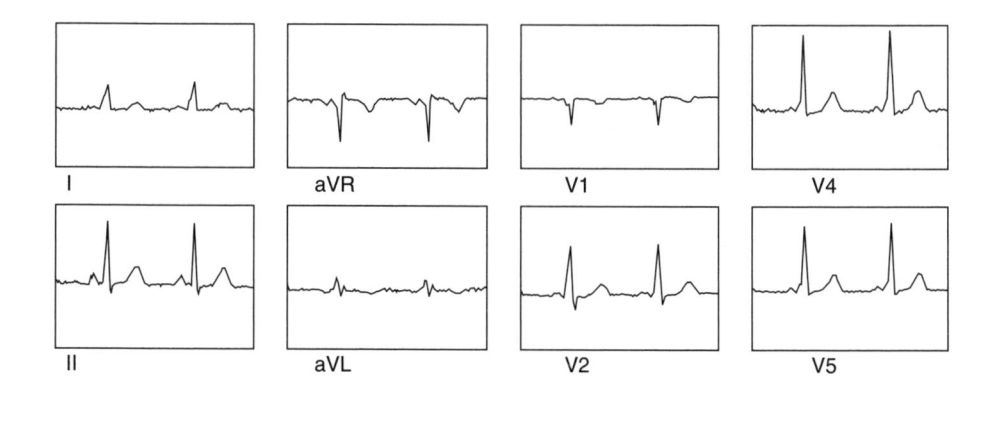

| I | aVR | V1 | V4 |
| II | aVL | V2 | V5 |

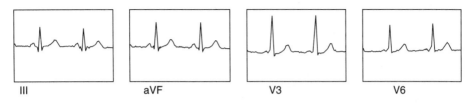

**Figure 6-7** • Wolff-Parkinson-White (WPW) syndrome. In this 12-lead ECG note the short PR interval and characteristic delta wave, which causes slurring at the onset of the QRS complex. The delta wave is best seen in leads $V_3$ to $V_6$.

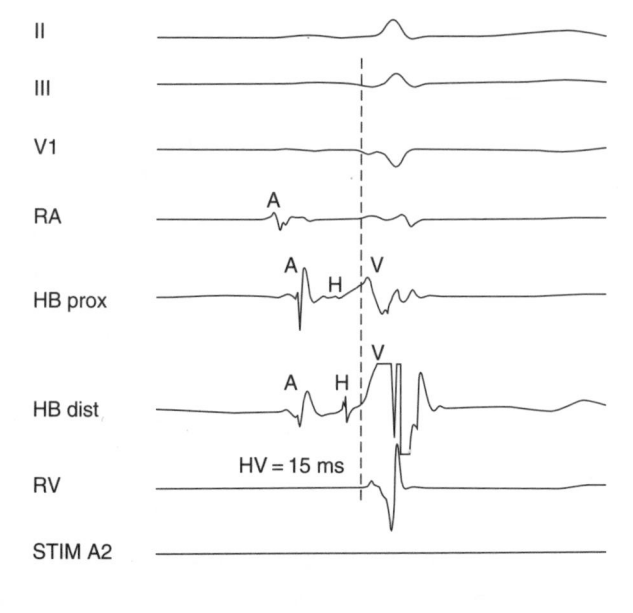

| II |
| III |
| V1 |
| RA |
| HB prox |
| HB dist |
| RV |
| STIM A2 |

A

A H V

A H V

HV = 15 ms

**Figure 6-8** • Shortened HV interval characteristic of an accessory pathway causing ventricular preexcitation. Shown are recordings from surface leads II, III, and V₁ and intracardiac recordings from the right atrium (RA), proximal and distal His bundle regions (HB prox, HB distal), and right ventricle (RV). The HV interval measured from the His bundle deflection to the onset of the QRS was 15 ms. The lower limit of normal for an HV interval is 35 ms. A, H, V = atrial, His bundle, and ventricular electrograms.

## Diagnosing the Presence of an Accessory Pathway

Overt accessory pathways are diagnosed by demonstrating ventricular preexcitation, which is often seen on the surface ECG by finding the characteristic delta waves of the WPW syndrome (Figure 6–7). On intracardiac recordings, a shortened HV interval (<35 ms) is seen (Figure 6–10A). Some patients have what is called latent preexcitation. In these patients the 12-lead ECG appears essentially normal without clear-cut delta waves, and their baseline HV interval is normal or only minimally shortened. The presence of ventricular preexcitation can be brought out by atrial overdrive pacing. This maneuver delays conduction across the AV node but not the accessory pathway, and it results in more ventricular activation via the accessory pathway with subsequent HV interval shortening and QRS complex widening (Figure 6–10B). Latent preexcitation can also be induced by giving agents that slow or block AV node conduction. The easiest agent to give is adenosine, which often causes transient complete AV nodal block and allows accessory pathway conduction to become manifest.

A concealed accessory pathway can be diagnosed by analyzing the pattern of atrial activation during ventricular pacing. The main diagnostic feature is eccentric atrial activation. Eccentric activation is said to be present when the atrium is activated earliest at a site other than the AV nodal region (Figure 6–11). In most patients its presence is fairly easy to confirm using a coronary sinus catheter to map the mitral annulus and a deflectable tip catheter to map the tricuspid annulus. In some patients, when the accessory pathway is located near the AV node the diagnosis is more difficult and other diagnostic maneuvers may be necessary.

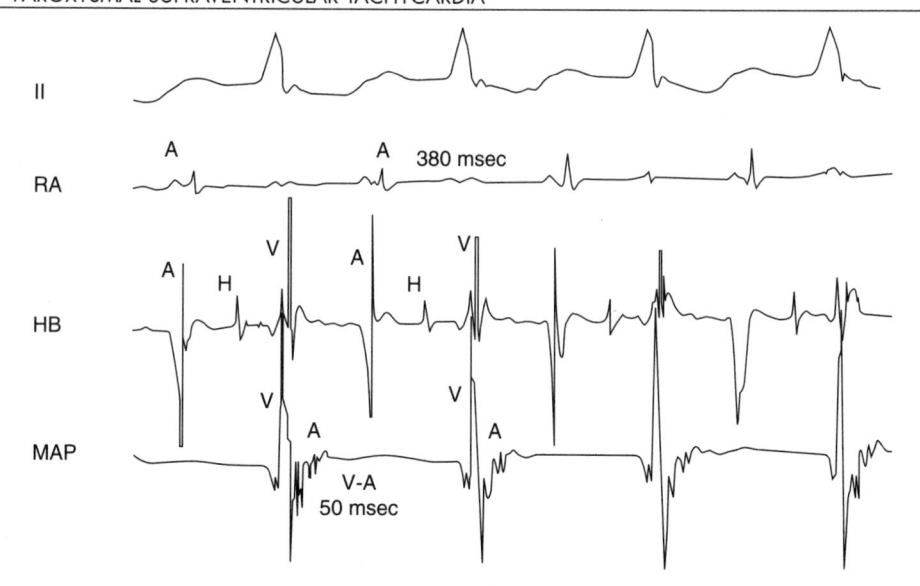

**Figure 6–9** • Atrial and ventricular ECG fusion when recordings were made near the accessory pathway during accessory pathway conduction. The ECGs were recorded during an episode of orthodromic reciprocating tachycardia. Shown are a recording from surface lead II and intracardiac recordings from the right atrium (RA), His bundle region (HB), and a mapping catheter (MAP) positioned in the left ventricle along the lateral mitral annulus. The tachycardia had a cycle length of 380 ms. Note that on the mapping catheter the ventricular (V) and atrial (A) electrograms are fused. This electrogram fusion is a result of the rapid conduction that occurs across most accessory pathways. A radiofrequency application at this mapping spot resulted in successful ablation of the accessory pathway.

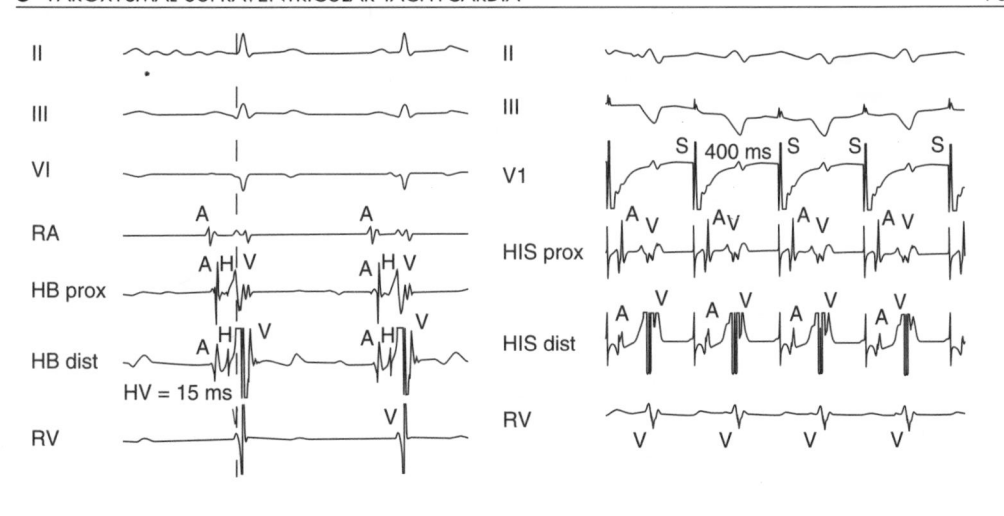

**Figure 6-10** • Ventricular preexcitation Wolff-Parkinson-White (WPW) syndrome. Shown are recordings from surface leads II, III, and $V_1$ and intracardiac recordings from the right atrium (RA), proximal and distal His bundle region (HB prox, HB dist), and right ventricle (RV). **(A)** Baseline recordings. There is a prominent His deflection on the His bundle distal electrogram, and the HV interval measured 15 ms, indicating the presence of ventricular preexcitation. **(B)** Atrial overdrive pacing (S) was performed at a cycle length of 400 ms. Note on the surface leads that there is increased widening of the QRS complex; and on the His bundle distal recording the His deflection is no longer visible and is buried in the ventricular electrogram (V). These changes are the result of an increase in the degree of ventricular preexcitation that occurs with more rapid atrial rates. This finding is characteristic of the WPW syndrome.

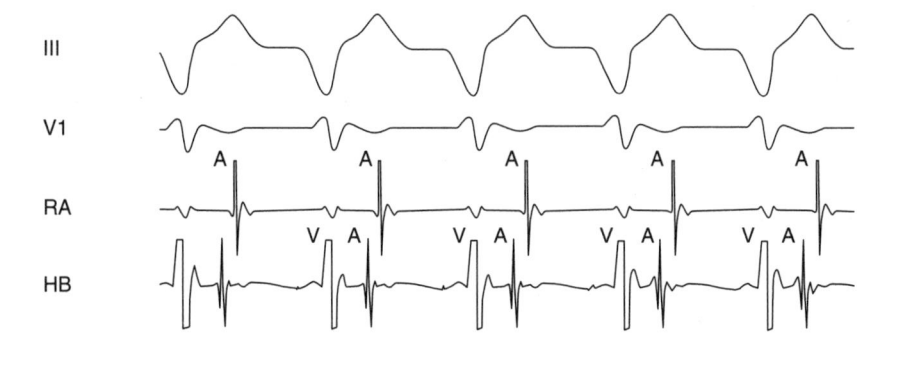

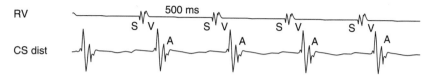

**Figure 6–11 •** Eccentric activation. Shown are recordings from surface leads III and V₁ and intracardiac recordings from the right atrium (RA), His bundle region (HB), right ventricle (RV), and distal coronary sinus (CS dist). Ventricular pacing (S) was performed at a cycle length of 500 ms. The earliest site of atrial activation was recorded on the CS distal catheter followed by that on the His bundle catheter and the right atrial catheter. Finding a site of atrial activation earlier than that in the His bundle region during VA conduction is termed eccentric activation and it is diagnostic of the presence of an accessory pathway. A, V = atrial and ventricular electrograms.

## Orthodromic Reciprocating Tachycardia

Orthodromic reciprocating tachycardia is an AV reentrant tachycardia that is the result of antegrade conduction down the AV node and retrograde conduction through the accessory pathway (Figure 6–1). Because antegrade conduction is via the normal His-Purkinje system, it usually results in a narrow complex tachycardia unless bundle branch aberration is present. In patients with known overt preexcitation (WPW syndrome), the occurrence of a narrow complex tachycardia is almost always due to ORT.

The major electrophysiologic feature of ORT is eccentric activation of the atrium with a short VA time recorded along either the mitral or tricuspid annulus during tachycardia. Prior to formal mapping of the annuli, the presence of ORT is suspected after finding a relatively long VA time (>90 ms) on the His bundle recording catheter (Figure 6–12). This long VA time is a direct result of eccentric activation of the atrium because it takes time for the impulse to spread from its initial point of activation across the atrium to the His bundle region. When a patient with PSVT is found to have a relatively long VA time at the His bundle region during tachycardia, formal mapping of the mitral and tricuspid annulus should be undertaken to look for the presence of eccentric activation. Patients with accessory pathways located in the anteroseptal and midseptal regions close to the AV node can be difficult to differentiate from AVNRT as they often have relatively short VA times (60–90 ms) and appear to have concentric activation of the atrium. These patients require additional pacing maneuvers to define the mechanism of the tachycardia. The characteristic features of ORT are summarized in Table 6–1.

## Ventricular Pacing During Orthodromic Reciprocating Tachycardia

As with AVNRT, ventricular overdrive pacing during ORT should result in entrainment of the tachycardia, assuming it does not terminate it (Figure 6–13). This pacing maneuver is especially helpful for differentiating ORT from atrial tachycardias. Atrial tachycardias, like ORTs, often have a long VA interval measured at the His bundle region. If entrainment is seen with ventricular overdrive pacing during tachycardia, it rules out an atrial tachycardia, and ORT should be strongly suspected.

Single ventricular extrastimuli delivered during tachycardia can also be helpful for establishing the presence of an accessory pathway. If an extrastimulus is placed at a time when the His bundle is refractory and the subsequent atrial depolarization of the tachycardia is advanced, an accessory pathway must be present (Figure 6–14). This is true because if the His bundle is refractory a ventricular impulse could not conduct retrograde through the His bundle–AV node axis, and the only way it could conduct to the atrium is via an accessory bypass tract. Although helpful, this pacing technique is usually not necessary to diagnose most cases of ORT. It can be helpful in confusing cases, such as tachycardias involving accessory pathways located in the anteroseptal or midseptal regions near the AV node, which are difficult to differentiate from AVNRT.

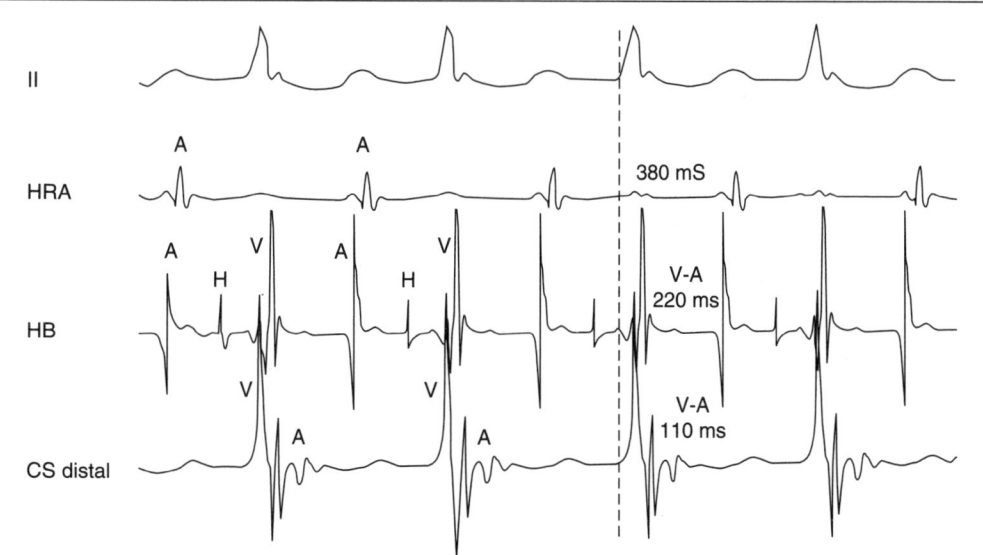

II

HRA

A    A    380 mS

HB

A    V    A    V    V-A
H        H        220 ms

V    V

CS distal

A    A    V-A
110 ms

**Figure 6-12** • Orthodromic reciprocating tachycardia (ORT). These tracings were recorded from a patient with a concealed left lateral accessory pathway during ORT with a cycle length of 380 ms. Shown are the recording from surface lead II and intracardiac recordings from the high right atrium (HRA), His bundle region (HB), and distal coronary sinus (CS distal). Eccentric activation of the atrium was seen with the earliest site of atrial activation noted on the CS distal catheter (VA = 110 ms). The HB catheter recorded a fairly late atrial activation time of 220 ms. Prior to formal mapping, a long VA time (≥100 ms) on the HB recordings suggests that an accessory pathway tachycardia may be present. A, V, H = atrial, ventricular, and His bundle electrograms.

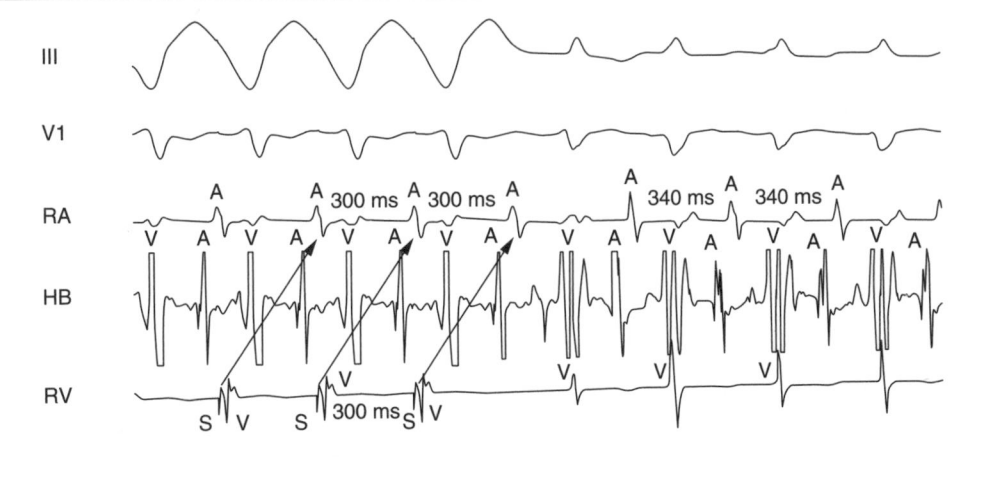

**Figure 6-13** • Entrainment of orthodromic reciprocating tachycardia (ORT). Shown are recordings from surface leads III and $V_1$ and intracardiac recordings from the right atrium (RA), His bundle region (HB), and right ventricle (RV). The patient was in tachycardia at a cycle length of 340 ms. Ventricular overdrive pacing (S) at a cycle length of 300 ms was performed and accelerated the atrial rate to the ventricular pacing rate. Upon termination of pacing, the tachycardia resumed at its previous rate and VA timing relations. This type of response to ventricular pacing essentially rules out an atrial tachycardia. A, V = atrial and ventricular electrograms.

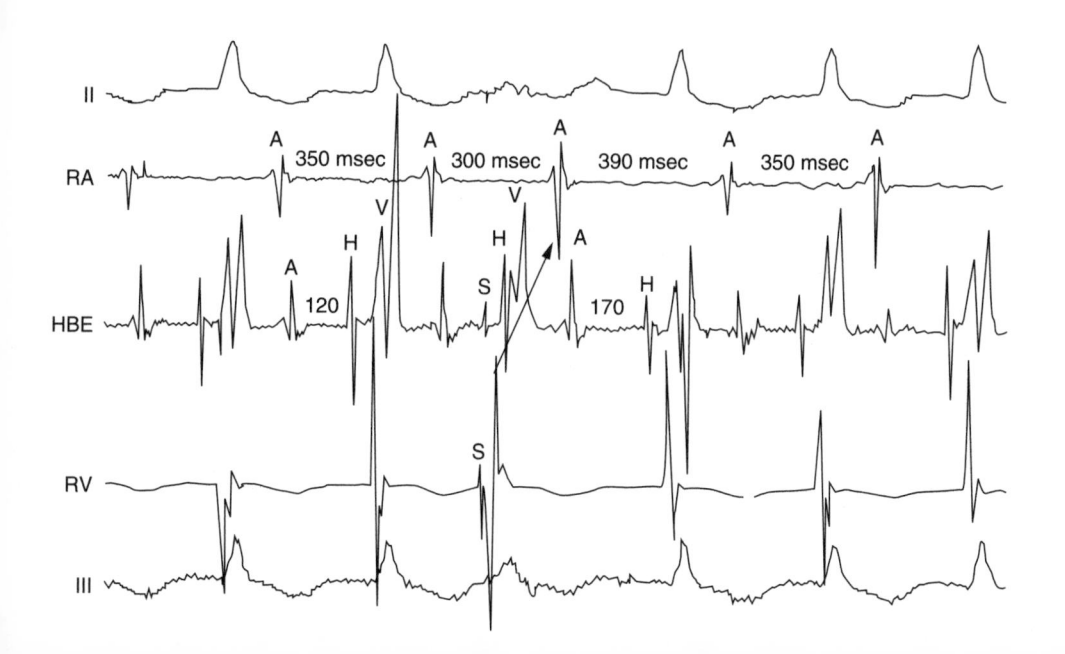

**Figure 6-14** • Atrial preexcitation. These tracings show the response of a patient in orthodromic reciprocating tachycardia (ORT) to the delivery of a single premature ventricular extrastimulus. Shown are recordings from surface leads II and III and intracardiac recordings from the right atrium (RA), His bundle region (HBE), and right ventricle (RV). The patient was in tachycardia at a cycle length of 350 ms. A ventricular extrastimulus (S) was delivered at a time when the His bundle was refractory because of antegrade activation from the tachycardia. The subsequent atrial depolarization was advanced (preexcited) and pulled in to a coupling interval of 300 ms. The only way for a ventricular extrastimulus to advance a subsequent atrial beat when the His bundle is refractory is via conduction across an accessory pathway. A, V, H = atrial, ventricular, and His bundle electrograms.

## ATRIAL TACHYCARDIA

Atrial tachycardias are the least common form of PSVT. The circuit or focus of an atrial tachycardia is localized completely in the atrium (Figure 6-1). Unlike AVNRT or ORT, atrial tachycardias are not dependent on antegrade conduction through the AV node or retrograde conduction through the AV node or an accessory pathway; therefore variable AV and VA times are often seen. When variable timing is seen during a PSVT, atrial tachycardia should be strongly suspected (Figure 6-15). Because AV conduction is not required, AV block can occur during an atrial tachycardia and not terminate the tachycardia (Figure 6-15). AV block always terminates ORT; it can occur with AVNRT when the region of block is below the AVNRT

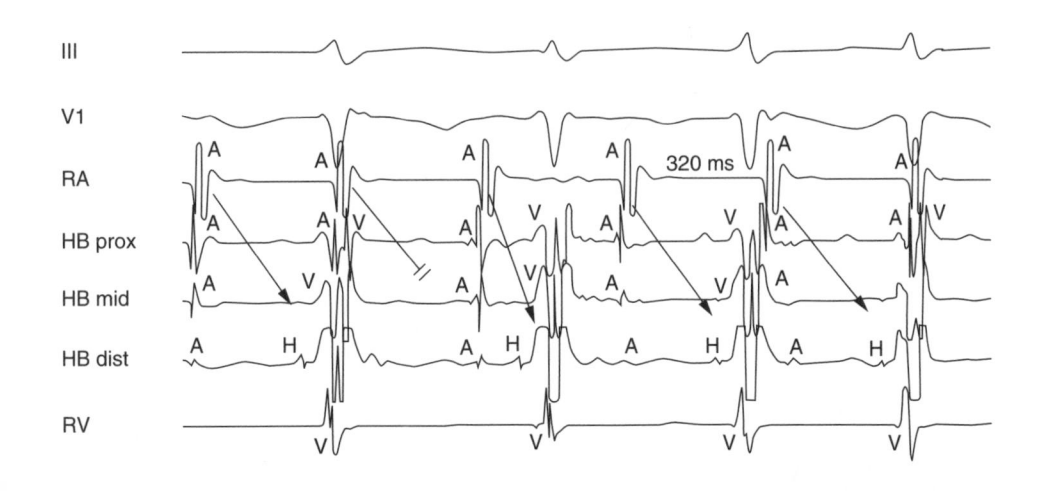

**Figure 6-15** • Atrial tachycardia. These recordings are from a patient with an atrial tachycardia with an atrial cycle length of 320 ms. Shown are recordings from surface leads III and $V_1$ and intracardiac recordings from the right atrium (RA), the proximal, mid, and distal His bundle regions (HB prox, HB mid, HB dist), and the right ventricle (RV). Note that during tachycardia there is AV block. The presence of AV block with continuation of the tachycardia rules out the possibility of an accessory pathway tachycardia. Also during tachycardia there is marked variability in the VA timing, making the possibility of AV node reentrant tachycardia much less likely and atrial tachycardia the probable diagnosis. A, V, H = atrial, ventricular, and His bundle electrograms.

---

circuit but is not particularly common. If entrainment with ventricular overdrive pacing is seen during tachycardia, it essentially rules out an atrial tachycardia but does not help differentiate between AVNRT or ORT. Probably the most helpful feature for differentiating an atrial tachycardia from the other two forms of PSVT is the atrial activation sequence during tachycardia. Atrial tachycardias can occur anywhere in the left or right atrium; therefore the earliest site of atrial activation during tachycardia is usually not at the AV node region or along the mitral or tricuspid annulus, as with AVNRT or ORT, respectively. Atrial tachycardias often arise in the more superior parts of the right or left atrium, resulting in a "high to low" activation sequence of the atrium. This "high to low" activation sequence is usually first noted by finding high right atrial activation occurring before atrial activation at the AV node region (Figure 6–16). When this pattern of atrial activation is seen, an atrial tachycardia should be strongly suspected and more formal atrial mapping performed.

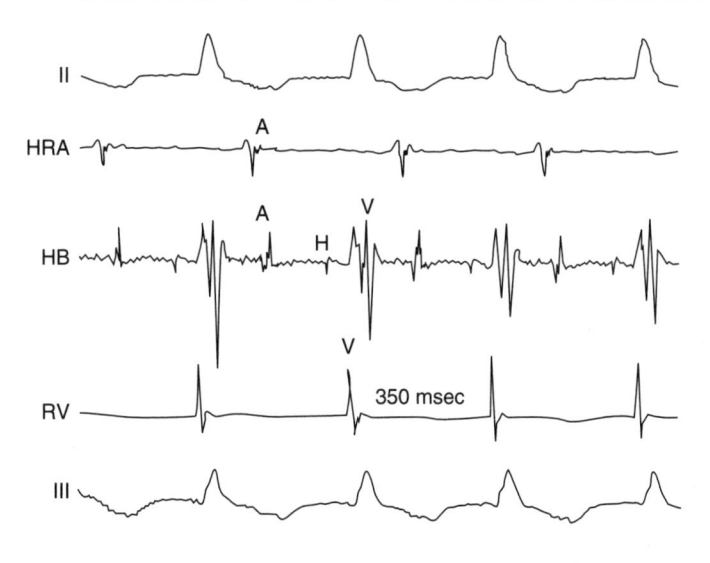

**Figure 6-16** • Atrial tachycardia. These tracings are from a patient with an atrial tachycardia arising in the right atrium along the superior portion of the lateral wall. Shown are recordings from surface leads II and III and intracardiac recordings from the high right atrium (HRA), His bundle region (HB), and right ventricle (RV). The tachycardia had a cycle length of 350 ms with 1:1 AV conduction. Note that atrial activation (A) in the high right atrium occurred before atrial activation at the His bundle region. This is called a "high to low" activation pattern and is most consistent with atrial tachycardia. The presence of atrial activation in the high right atrium before the His bundle region essentially rules out an AV node reentrant tachycardia or orthodromic reciprocating tachycardia (ORT) using a left-sided accessory pathway. ORT with a right-sided accessory pathway is still a possibility, and mapping the tricuspid annulus along with pacing maneuvers should be performed to evaluate for this possibility. A, V, H = atrial, ventricular, and His bundle electrograms.

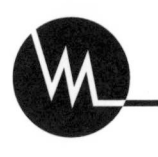

# VENTRICULAR TACHYCARDIA

The purpose of this chapter is to outline the electrophysiologist's approach to the diagnosis and treatment of ventricular tachycardia so others working with these patients can better anticipate the type of evaluation required. Ventricular tachycardia is most frequently recognized as a wide QRS complex tachycardia on the electrocardiogram (ECG). Patients may be asymptomatic or have symptoms ranging from mild palpitations to syncope or hemodynamic collapse. In this chapter we review the underlying physiology of ventricular tachycardia, the ECG and electrophysiologic diagnosis of ventricular tachycardia, and the various types of ventricular tachycardia along with the therapeutic options available for treatment.

## PHYSIOLOGY

There are three major physiologic mechanisms that govern the initiation and maintenance of ventricular tachycardias: abnormal automaticity, reentry, and triggered activity.

## Abnormal Automaticity

Ventricular tachycardias caused by abnormal automaticity are often polymorphic with beat-to-beat variability in QRS morphology (Figure 7–1A). They often have a characteristic "warm up/cool down" rate behavior, meaning that there is a gradual increase and decrease in the heart rate at the initiation and termination of the tachycardia. These tachycardias are usually provoked by metabolic changes, such as ischemia and electrolyte imbalance: they are generally not induced by ventricular programmed stimulation during electrophysiologic testing.

## Reentry

Reentrant ventricular tachycardias are characteristically monomorphic (uniform beat-to-beat QRS morphology) (Figure 7–1B) and usually have an abrupt onset and termination. The reentrant circuit is frequently the result of an anatomic abnormality, most often myocardial scarring from coronary artery disease. These tachycardias are often inducible with ventricular programmed stimulation during electrophysiologic testing.

## Triggered Activity

Ventricular tachycardia caused by triggered activity is characterized by a monomorphic appearance and a rate behavior that demonstrates a warm up/cool down phenomenon. It is often initiated by adrenergic stimuli such as an isoproterenol infusion and often terminates with an infusion of calcium channel blocking

A

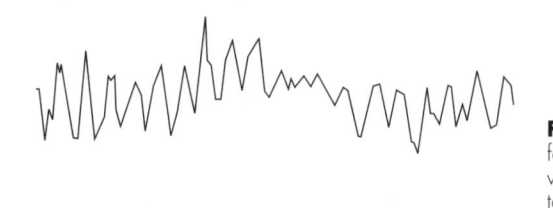

B

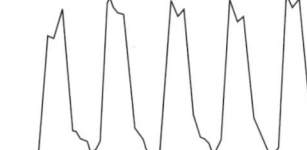

**Figure 7–1 • (A)** Characteristic surface ECG appearance of polymorphic ventricular tachycardia. Note the beat-to-beat variation in QRS morphology. **(B)** Characteristic appearance of monomorphic ventricular tachycardia. Note the nearly identical beat-to-beat appearance of the QRS morphology.

agent or adenosine. Triggered ventricular tachycardia can often be induced with overdrive ventricular pacing or programmed ventricular stimulation during electrophysiologic testing.

## ELECTROCARDIOGRAPHIC AND ELECTROPHYSIOLOGIC EVALUATION OF VENTRICULAR TACHYCARDIA

A common dilemma associated with the ECG diagnosis of ventricular tachycardia is differentiating it from supraventricular tachycardia with aberrancy. The ECG criteria that may be helpful for confirming a diagnosis of ventricular tachycardia include the following:

• Atrioventricular dissociation
• QRS duration >140 ms
• Atypical right or left bundle branch block patterns
• Extreme axis deviation
• Positive concordance of the precordial leads
• Capture or fusion beats

Unfortunately, a 12-lead ECG is not often obtained, and only a rhythm strip may be available. In such cases reproduction of the wide complex tachycardia during an electrophysiology study can often confirm or refute the diagnosis of ventricular tachycardia.

The electrophysiologic induction of ventricular tachycardia is usually achieved by programmed stimulation of the right ventricle. During programmed ventricular stimulation a drive train of eight pacing impulses is delivered followed by a variable number of extrastimuli (usually one to four) (Figure 7–2). The pacing outputs in the eight-beat drive train are referred to as S1, and the extrastimuli are referred to as S2, S3, and S4 for the first, second, and third extrastimuli, respectively. The coupling intervals between the drive train and the extrastimuli are progressively shortened until there is failure of the first extrastimulus to capture (ventricular refractoriness). Programmed stimulation is usually performed from at least two right ventricular sites using three basic drive train cycle lengths and up to four extrastimuli. Straight burst pacing of the ventricle without extrastimulation is also employed to induce ventricular tachycardia. Two of the most commonly used ventricular stimulation protocols are outlined in Table 7–1.

Figure 7–3 shows a typical rhythm strip of a wide complex tachycardia that could be either ventricular tachycardia or supraventricular tachycardia with aberrancy. Note that with reproduction of this tachycardia during an electrophysiology study there is atrioventricular (AV) dissociation noted in the intracardiac recordings (Figure 7–4). There is also loss of the His bundle electrogram preceding every QRS, confirming that it was not a supraventricular tachycardia. Most supraventricular tachycardias demonstrate a His bundle electrogram preceding every QRS due to their obligatory conduction from the atria to the ventricle via the AV node and His bundle.

Sometimes single ventricular beats or short runs of nonsustained ventricular tachycardia are induced during programmed ventricular stimulation. Generally, the induced ventricular tachycardia must meet the following criteria to be considered a clinically relevant finding:

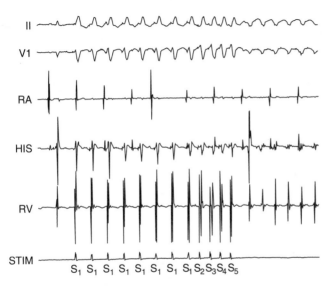

**Figure 7–2** • Typical delivery of an eight-beat drive train of ventricular stimuli ($S_1$), followed by four extrastimuli that are closely coupled ($S_2$, $S_3$, $S_4$, and $S_5$) with subsequent initiation of sustained monomorphic ventricular tachycardia. Recordings are from surface leads II and $V_1$. RA = right atrial electrogram; HIS = His bundle electrogram; RV = right ventricular electrogram; STIM = right ventricular pacing stimuli.

## Table 7-1 COMMONLY USED VENTRICULAR STIMULATION PROTOCOLS

| | 18-STEP PROTOCOL | | | 6-STEP PROTOCOL | | |
|---|---|---|---|---|---|---|
| STEP | SITE* | BDCL | ES | SITE* | BDCL | BDCL |
| 1 | 1 | 350 | 1 | 1 | 350 | 4 |
| 2 | 1 | 350 | 2 | 1 | 400 | 4 |
| 3 | 1 | 350 | 3 | 1 | 600 | 4 |
| 4 | 1 | 400 | 1 | 2 | 350 | 4 |
| 5 | 1 | 400 | 2 | 2 | 400 | 4 |
| 6 | 1 | 400 | 3 | 2 | 600 | 4 |
| 7 | 1 | 600 | 1 | | | |
| 8 | 1 | 600 | 2 | | | |
| 9 | 1 | 600 | 3 | | | |
| 10 | 2 | 350 | 1 | | | |
| 11 | 2 | 350 | 2 | | | |
| 12 | 2 | 350 | 3 | | | |
| 13 | 2 | 400 | 1 | | | |
| 14 | 2 | 400 | 2 | | | |
| 15 | 2 | 400 | 3 | | | |
| 16 | 2 | 600 | 1 | | | |
| 17 | 2 | 600 | 2 | | | |
| 18 | 2 | 600 | 3 | | | |

BDCL = basic drive cycle length (in milliseconds); ES = number of extrastimuli.
*Step 1 is the right ventricular apex; site 2 is the right ventricular outflow tract or septum.

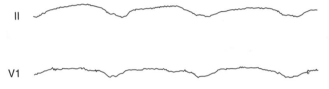

**Figure 7-3** • Typical appearance of monomorphic ventricular tachycardia from two surface ECG leads: II and $V_1$.

II

V1

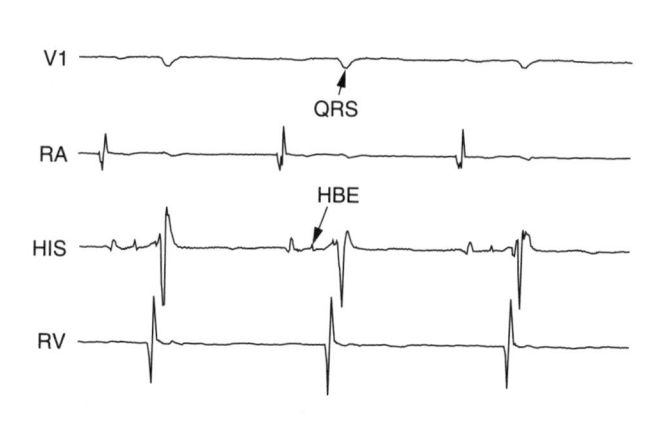

**Figure 7-4 • (A)** Intracardiac and surface ECG recordings of normal sinus rhythm. There are intracardiac recordings from the right atrium (RA), His bundle (HIS), and right ventricle (RV). Surface ECG recordings are from leads II and $V_1$. Note the appearance of a His bundle spike (HBE) preceding every QRS.

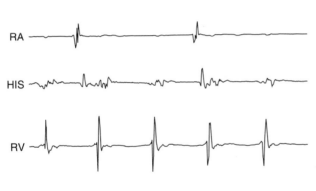

B

II

V1

RA

HIS

RV

**Figure 7-4 • (B)** Intracardiac tracing during ventricular tachycardia in the same patient as in Figure 7-3. Note the dissociation between the right ventricular intracardiac electrogram (RV) and the right atrial intracardiac electrogram (RA). Note also the disappearance of the His bundle electrogram (HIS) preceding every QRS on the His channel recording compared to Figure 7-4A.

- Duration of >30 seconds
- Reproducible morphology
- Cycle length ≥ 240 ms or more

Polymorphic ventricular tachycardia and ventricular fibrillation are generally considered nonspecific findings and are not reliable endpoints during electrophysiologic testing.

## TYPES OF VENTRICULAR TACHYCARDIA

The underlying physiology of the ventricular tachycardia is often diagnosed by its ECG appearance and its behavior during electrophysiology testing. The most common types of monomorphic and polymorphic ventricular tachycardia are outlined below.

### Monomorphic Ventricular Tachycardias

Reentrant Ventricular Tachycardia

Slow conduction from myocardial scar provides the usual substrate for reentry. Electrophysiologic testing induces sustained monomorphic ventricular tachycardia in more than 90% of patients with a history of coronary disease and sustained ventricular tachycardia. The treatment options include electrophysiologically guided antiarrhythmic therapy, an implantable cardioverter-defibrillator, or radiofrequency ablation (if hemodynamically well tolerated). Pharmacologic therapy is considered successful if a reproducibly inducible ventricular tachycardia is rendered noninducible on antiarrhythmic therapy at follow-up electrophysiologic testing or if the tachycardia is converted from a hemodynamically unstable to a hemodynamically stable arrhythmia.

## Bundle Branch Reentrant Ventricular Tachycardias

Bundle branch reentrant ventricular tachycardias occur in the setting of ischemic or nonischemic dilated cardiomyopathies with associated His-Purkinje conduction disease. The substrate for reentry is a conduction system with enough disease to allow unidirectional block and reentry (Figure 7–5). The ECG morphology is usually left bundle superior axis (Figure 7–6), and the baseline ECG usually demonstrates an intraventricular conduction delay (Figure 7–7). The electrophysiology study allows recognition of bundle branch reentrant ventricular tachycardia through characteristic HV prolongation at baseline, a His bundle electrogram preceding each QRS complex of the ventricular tachycardia with prolongation of the HV interval during tachycardia over the baseline HV interval (Figure 7–7), and changes in the His–His interval preceding any change in the subsequent RR intervals. The treatment of choice in this form of ventricular tachycardia is bundle branch ablation, often coupled with an implantable defibrillator implant.

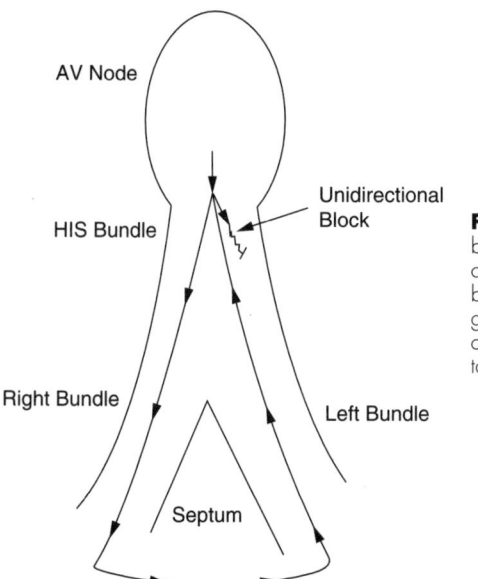

**Figure 7-5** • Conduction delay and subsequent block in the left bundle branch. The path of electrical depolarization then proceeds down the right bundle, across the ventricular septum, and retrogradely up the left bundle to create a reentrant circuit typical of bundle branch reentrant ventricular tachycardia.

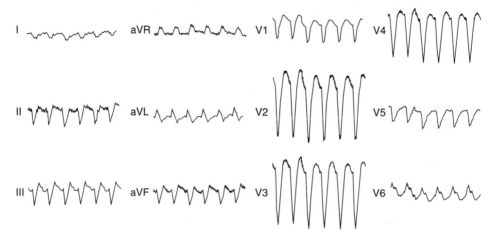

**Figure 7-6 •** This tracing of ventricular tachycardia represents the typical appearance of bundle branch re-entrant tachycardia. Note the terminal S wave in lead V$_1$ (confirming the left bundle branch morphology) and the negative QRS deflections in leads II, III, and aVF, indicating an overall direction of electrical propagation away from the inferior wall (confirming a superior axis).

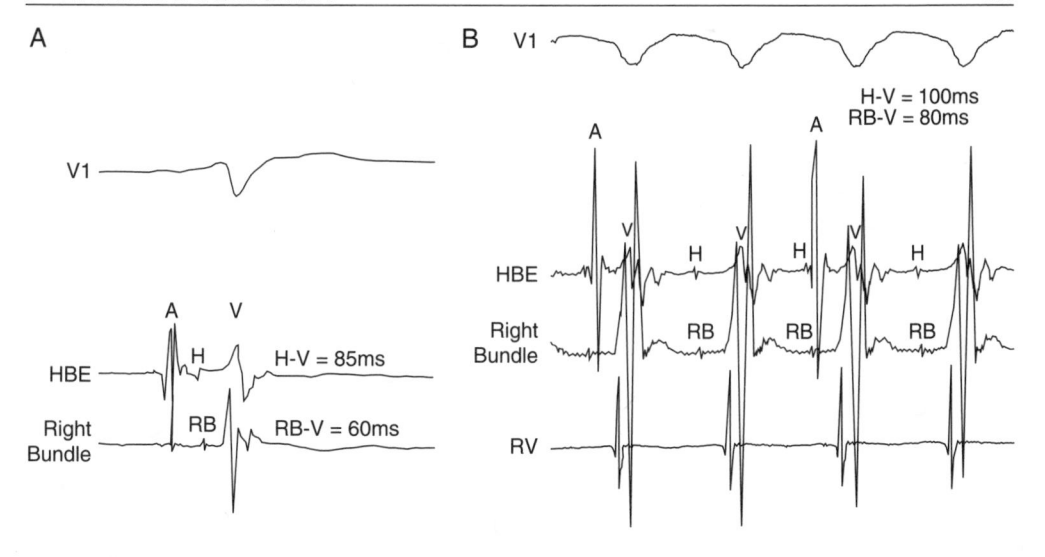

**Figure 7-7 • (A)** This surface and intracardiac electrogram tracing demonstrates the baseline prolongation of conduction from the His bundle (H) and right bundle (RB) to the ventricle (V) via prolonged H-V and RB-V conduction times. The surface tracing is from lead $V_1$. HBE = intracardiac recording from the His bundle; RB = recording of the right bundle electrogram from the endocardium of the right ventricle; A = recording of an intraatrial electrogram on the HBE channel. **(B)** This tracing is a surface ECG and intracardiac recordings after the onset of bundle branch reentrant ventricular tachycardia in the same patient depicted in normal sinus rhythm in 7-7A. Note the prolongation in His bundle-to-ventricular conduction and right bundle-to-ventricular conduction after the onset of the tachycardia compared to the baseline normal sinus rhythm. $V_1$ represents an ECG recording from the surface lead $V_1$. HBE represents an intracardiac recording from the His bundle; and RV indicates an intracardiac recording from the right ventricle.

## Idiopathic Monomorphic Ventricular Tachycardia

Idiopathic monomorphic ventricular tachycardias are usually a manifestation of triggered activity and often occur in structurally normal hearts. The surface 12-lead ECG or rhythm strip demonstrates a warm-up rate phenomenon with a left bundle inferior axis morphology for triggered activity from the right ventricular outflow tract (RV outflow tract VT) (Figure 7–8) and a right bundle superior axis when the triggered activity is from the left ventricle (idiopathic LV VT) (Figure 7–9). During electrophysiologic testing the tachycardias are induced with burst pacing or, less commonly, with programmed stimulation. The tachycardia is usually easily reproducible but not always sustainable; it often requires catecholamine provocation with isoproterenol for induction. The drive cycle length of burst pacing usually affects the cycle length of the induced ventricular tachycardia, and the induction is often site-specific. Treatment options include β-blocker or calcium channel blocker therapy (which varies in its effectiveness) or catheter ablation (with greater than 90% success if induction of the clinical tachycardia is achieved). Magnetic resonance imaging (MRI) is often required prior to ablation of right ventricular tachycardias to rule out the possibility of arrhythmogenic right ventricular dysplasia, which confers a high risk of myocardial perforation during the ablation procedure.

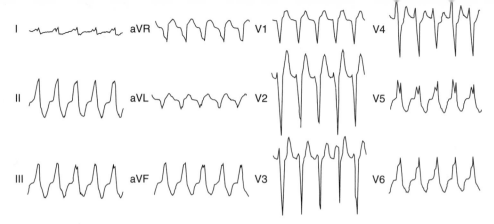

**Figure 7-8** • This tracing depicts a typical surface ECG recording of right ventricular outflow tract ventricular tachycardia. Note the negative deflection in the terminal portion of the QRS complex in lead $V_1$, indicating left bundle morphology. Note the overall upward deflection of the QRS complex in the inferior leads (surface leads II, III, and aVF), which indicates an overall direction of electrical propagation toward the inferior wall of the heart (an inferior axis).

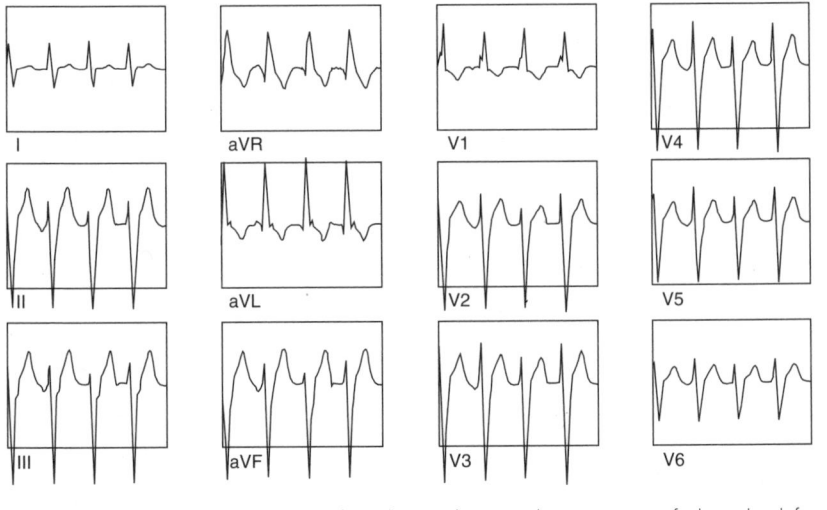

**Figure 7-9 •** This 12-lead surface ECG recording depicts the typical appearance of idiopathic left ventricular tachycardia. Note the wide rsR configuration of the QRS complex in lead $V_1$, indicating right bundle morphology. Also note the superior axis of electrical propagation with a negative deflection of the QRS complex in the inferior leads II, III, and aVF.

## Polymorphic Ventricular Tachycardias

Polymorphic ventricular tachycardia is an unstable ventricular arrhythmia with beat-to-beat QRS morphology variation. Patients who present with polymorphic ventricular tachycardia can be classified into those with a normal baseline QT interval and those with a prolonged QT interval. This ECG characteristic helps separate these patients based on underlying pathophysiologic substrate.

### Patients with a Long QT Interval at Baseline

Patients with a long QT interval at baseline (QTc > 440 ms) and polymorphic ventricular tachycardia usually suffer from acquired or congenital long-QT syndrome. Acquired long-QT syndrome is caused by abnormal after-depolarizations, and the initiation of polymorphic ventricular tachycardia is usually preceded by a significant bradycardia or a long pause such as that found during complete heart block (Figure 7–10). Among the most common causative pharmacologic agents are class 1A and III antiarrhythmic agents: phenothiazines and tricyclic antidepressants. Hypomagnesemia or hypokalemia, intrinsic bradyarrhythmias, and liquid protein diets can also be causative. Treatment involves removal or correction of underlying causes, infusion of catecholamines and intravenous magnesium, overdrive ventricular pacing, or a combination of these methods.

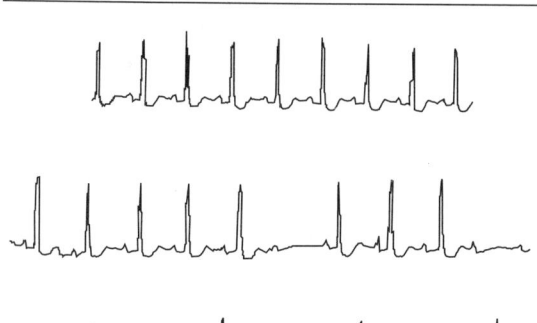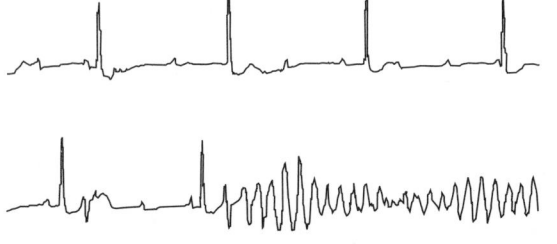

**Figure 7-10** • This tracing represents the typical pause-dependent onset of polymorphic ventricular tachycardia during complete heart block.

Congenital long-QT syndrome is thought to be caused by abnormal after-depolarizations, but polymorphic ventricular tachycardia is usually initiated during enhanced adrenergic tone (emotional upset, exertional stress). These patients can suffer initiation of an arrhythmic event at any time and may have a normal QT interval at baseline with the only hint of pathology being a family history of sudden cardiac death. The abnormal repolarization patterns are often elicited by intravenous infusions of isoproterenol or are discovered during stress testing or Holter monitoring. Electrophysiologic testing is generally not helpful, and treatment involves β-blockers, sympathectomy, permanent pacing, or implantable cardioverter-defibrillator placement.

## Patients with a Normal QT Interval at Baseline

Patients with polymorphic ventricular tachycardia, no evidence of repolarization abnormalities on Holter monitoring or after infusion of catecholamines, and no family history of sudden death suffer from short-coupled torsades or short-coupled polymorphic ventricular tachycardia. The cause is usually cardiac ischemia, which causes abnormal automaticity. A nonischemic variety has also been described. The electrophysiology study can be diagnostic of the nonischemic variety if polymorphic ventricular tachycardia is induced during programmed ventricular stimulation at long coupling intervals. Treatment is confined to correction of the underlying ischemia, implantable defibrillator placement, and suppression with verapamil in combination with implantable defibrillator placement in idiopathic cases.

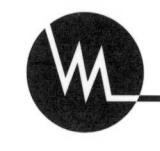

# CHAPTER 8

# EVALUATION AND MANAGEMENT OF SYNCOPE

Syncope is defined as a sudden, transient loss of consciousness associated with an inability to maintain an upright posture, with spontaneous recovery. It is a frequent symptom and accounts for approximately 3% of all emergency room visits and up to 6% of general hospital admissions in the United States. A wide variety of neurologic, cardiovascular, and metabolic disorders may result in syncope, as shown in Chart 8–1. The most common causes of syncope in the general population are neurocardiogenic syncope and those that are cardiovascularly related (arrhythmias and structural heart disease). These entities are evaluated by electrophysiologists and are discussed in detail later in the text.

## MORTALITY

Mortality after syncope depends on the underlying cause. The incidence of sudden death after a syncopal event with associated cardiovascular disease has been reported to range between 18% and 33% at 1 year. Patients without cardiovascular disease are at low risk for sudden death. Therefore it is important to identify the high risk patients so the risk of sudden death can hopefully be reduced.

## Chart 8-1
### CAUSES OF SYNCOPE

- Neuroautonomic regulation
  - Neurocardiogenic (vasodepressor) syncope
  - Situational
    - Cough syncope
    - Swallow syncope
    - Micturation syncope
    - Defecation syncope
    - Syncope associated with pain
  - Carotid sinus hypersensitivity syndrome
- Arrhythmias
  - Sinus node dysfunction
  - Atrioventricular block
  - Supraventricular tachycardia
  - Ventricular tachycardia
- Mechanical cardiovascular disease
  - Aortic stenosis
  - Mitral stenosis
  - Obstructive cardiomyopathy
  - Atrial myxoma
  - Severe pulmonary vascular disease
  - Prosthetic valve dysfunction
  - Cerebrovascular and neurologic
    - Vertebrobasilar transient ischemic attacks
    - Migraine
    - Subclavian steal syndrome
    - Seizure disorders
  - Orthostatic hypotension
    - Hypovolemia
    - Autonomic insufficiency

*continues*

**Chart 8-1**
CAUSES OF SYNCOPE *(Continued)*

- Drug-induced (commonly nitrates, β-blockers, and vasodilators)
    - Hypoglycemia
    - Hypoxia
    - Hyperventilation
- Psychiatric
    - Panic disorders
    - Hysteria
    - Conversion reaction
    - Malingering

## INITIAL EVALUATION

Initial evaluation of syncope includes a thorough history and physical examination, electrocardiogram (ECG), and evaluation of cardiac function after an echocardiogram. The history and physical examination comprise the cornerstone of the evaluation of syncope. They may reveal findings suggestive of specific entities as possible causes and may be helpful for determining the most appropriate initial diagnostic tests, if indicated.

A description regarding the syncopal event is obtained from the patient and any witness present. The following information should be solicited: the events leading to the episode, prodromal and residual symptoms, and the presence of injury secondary to the syncopal event. Physical examination findings that may be helpful are those related to orthostatic hypotension, abnormal cardiovascular findings, and neurologic abnormalities.

The ECG is primarily a marker for the presence of heart disease. Specific abnormalities that may lead to further direction for diagnostic testing include the presence of Q waves, bundle branch block, hypertrophy, ischemia, atrioventricular (AV) block, and Wolff-Parkinson-White syndrome. The echocardiogram provides additional information related to the presence of coronary artery disease, structural heart disease, cardiomyopathies, or vascular disease.

Carotid sinus massage can be performed during the physical examination to identify carotid hypersensitivity: cardioinhibitory and vasodepressor. Carotid massage is usually done in the presence of ECG and blood pressure monitoring to detect both cardioinhibitory and vasodepressor components of this problem. An abnormal response is defined as cardiac systole of more than 3–5 seconds or a systolic blood pressure decline of 50 mm Hg or more. Although carotid hypersensitivity is considered a rare cause of syncope, there are some circumstances in which this entity should be highly suspected: (1) when carotid sinus massage reproduces the patient's symptoms; and (2) when certain activities trigger the patient's spontaneous symptoms (e.g., turning the head, wearing a seat belt, shaving).

If the syncope is thought to be cardiovascularly related (structural heart disease, vasodepressor syncope, or cardiac arrhythmias), further testing may be indicated. Such additional evaluations include heart catheterization, tilt table testing, or electrophysiology testing.

As previously mentioned, patients with syncope and suspect cardiovascular disease are at high risk for sudden death and must be evaluated aggressively. These patients often require stress testing or heart catheterization to characterize their cardiovascular disease. Patients with underlying structural heart disease and syncope often necessitate an electrophysiology study to rule out serious arrhythmias as a cause of their syncope.

If the syncope is not associated with structural heart disease, further evaluation may include long-term ambulatory monitoring, treadmill testing, or tilt table testing. A flow diagram that summarizes the diagnostic approach to the evaluation of syncope is shown in Figure 8–1. The following sections describe in more detail the evaluation and management of syncope related to electrophysiology concerns: neurocardiogenic syncope and cardiac arrhythmias.

## NEUROCARDIOGENIC SYNCOPE

The mechanisms of neurocardiogenic syncope are still not fully understood. This entity has been identified by a variety of names (e.g., vasodepressor, vasovagal, situational) in an effort to describe the variants or possible causative mechanisms of syncope. Current theory suggests that with all variants of neurocardiogenic syncope the medullary vasodepressor region of the brain stem is stimulated via afferent pathways. Such stimulation results in inhibition of sympathetic tone and generation of efferent signals of increased vagal tone via the vagus nerve with subsequent hypotension.

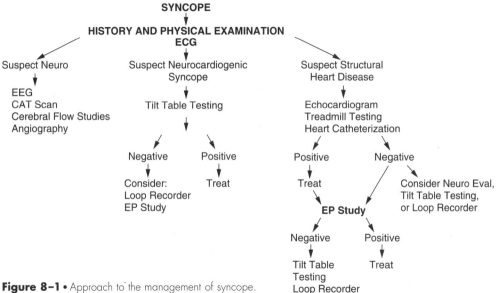

**Figure 8-1 •** Approach to the management of syncope.

Syncope that is neurocardiogenic in origin often exhibits characteristic features, listed in Chart 8–2. Neurocardiogenic syncope is occasionally presumed to be a seizure disorder. Compounding the problems with diagnosis is the occasional development of mild seizure-like movements during the neurocardiogenic syncopal event. They are the result of a temporary decrease in cerebral blood flow due to transient hypotension. As discussed previously, an in-depth review of the patient's episode of syncope may provide clues helpful during the diagnostic evaluation. Table 8–1 notes the distinguishing clinical features of neurocardiogenic syncope and neurologic seizure.

## Tilt Table Testing

In recent years tilt table testing has been used to evaluate the predisposition to neurocardiogenic syncope. The upright posture on the tilt table results in peripheral venous pooling, which decreases venous return to the heart. Reflex tachycardia and an increase in left ventricular pressure presumably stimulate cardiac C fibers, resulting in hypotension or bradycardia (or both), which have input into the vasodepressor region to activate the neurocardiogenic reflex. A tilt table is shown in Figure 8–2.

### Indications

The indications for tilt table testing have been outlined by the ACC Expert Consensus Document (published in the *Journal of American College of Cardiology*, 1996). They are summarized in Chart 8–3.

### Chart 8-2
NEUROCARDIOGENIC SYNCOPE: CLINICAL FEATURES

- Associated trigger mechanism
  - Upright posture, particularly prolonged standing
  - Pain (gastrointestinal, genitourinary)
  - Emotional upset
  - Fear or anxiety
  - After exercise
- Prodromal (warning) symptoms (may improve with sitting or lying down)
  - Nausea
  - Diaphoresis
  - Lightheadedness
- Pallor
- Palpitations
- Visual disturbances
- Resolution of syncopal event
  - Occurs almost immediately after lying or falling down
- Residual symptoms
  - Fatigue/weakness
  - Nausea
  - Diaphoresis
  - Headache

| Table 8-1 | DISTINGUISHING CLINICAL FEATURES OF NEUROCARDIOGENIC SYNCOPE AND NEUROLOGIC SEIZURE |
|---|---|
| Neurocardiogenic syncope | Neurologioc seizure |
| Face pale in color | Face bluish in color |
| Associated with "trigger" | Mouth frothing |
| Nausea and sweating before event | Tongue biting |
| Oriented after event | Disorientation after event |
| | Unconscious >5 minutes |
| | Incontinent |

## Laboratory Environment and Equipment

It is recommended that the tilt table test be performed with low level lighting and at a comfortable temperature. The equipment necessary includes a tilt table with safety straps that is capable of smooth, rapid transitions up to 90 degrees and down to a horizontal position. Other essentials include an ECG monitor/defibrillator with pacing capabilities, automatic blood pressure machine, manual blood pressure cuff, Doppler, intravenous (IV) infusion pump, IV supplies, emergency medications (atropine), and an admixture of 250 ml dextrose in water with 1 mg of isoproterenol (Isuprel) to be used for pharmacologic provocation. A standard emergency cart should be in the room or in close proximity to it.

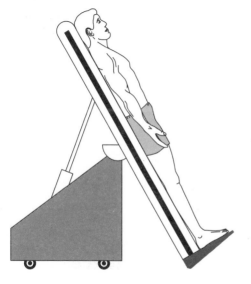

**Figure 8-2** • Tilt table.

**Chart 8–3**
**INDICATIONS FOR TILT TABLE TESTING**

*Tilt table testing is warranted*
- Recurrent syncope of unknown etiology
- Single syncopal episode in high risk patient with or without a history suggestive of neuro-cardiogenic syncope
- Evaluation of patients in whom neurocardiogenic syncope is suspected and would affect treatment plans
- Evaluation of exercise-induced or exercise-associated syncope
- Reasonable differences of opinion exist regarding the utility of tilt table testing

*Differentiating convulsive syncope from seizures*
- Assessing patients with recurrent unexplained falls
- Evaluating recurrent presyncope or dizziness

- Evaluating unexplained syncope with associated peripheral neuropathies or dysautonomias
- Follow-up to evaluate effectiveness of neurocardiogenic therapy

*Tilt table testing is not warranted*
- One episode of clear-cut vasovagal type syncope without injury
- Syncope of another identified cause and in which additional demonstration of cardiogenic syncope would not alter the plan of treatment

*Potential emerging indications*
- Recurrent idiopathic vertigo
- Recurrent transient ischemic attacks
- Chronic fatigue syndrome
- Sudden infant death syndrome

Patient Education and Preparation

The primary components of patient preparation for a tilt table test is to educate the patient about the need for the procedure and how it is performed, and to apply the protective and monitoring devices. Chart 8–4 reviews the educational points to be addressed with the patient.

Protocol

Controversy exists among physicians regarding various aspects of tilt table protocols. Major points of disagreement are the degree of the table angle, duration of the baseline (drug-free) tilt, and use of the pharmacologic provocative agents. The protocol suggested in Chart 8–5 is based on recommendations in the ACC Expert Consensus Document.

## Management of Patients with Neurocardiogenic Syncope

Management of patients with neurocardiogenic syncope includes patient education and counseling and pharmacologic therapy. Issues related to educating and counseling the patient with neurocardiogenic syncope are summarized in Chart 8–6.

Medications used to control neurocardiogenic syncope are effective owing to one of several mechanisms. β-Adrenergic blocking agents work by their negative inotropic action. Volume-expanding agents help maintain cardiac filling pressures. Vagolytic agents are useful for diminishing the efferent hypervago-

### Chart 8-4
PATIENT EDUCATION FOR TILT TABLE TESTING

- Review the mechanism of neurocardiogenic syncope and purpose of the tilt table test.
- Provide instructions regarding when to begin the preprocedure fasting state.
- Review the safety precautions that will be used during the test to prevent injury (safety strap).
- Discuss the importance of reporting symptoms and whether they are familiar to the staff during the test.
- Review the tilt table positions (up and down); reassure the patient that its positions change gradually and do not rotate.
- Discuss the monitoring equipment to be used during the procedure and its purpose (ECG and blood pressure cuffs).
- Discuss the need for an indwelling intravenous catheter and the short-term but potentially uncomfortable side effects of medication infusions.
- Instruct patient to have available transportation home after the procedure.
- Obtain consent for the procedure.

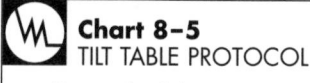

**Chart 8-5**
TILT TABLE PROTOCOL

- Quiet, dim laboratory
- Supine equilibration period of 20–45 minutes
- NPO overnight or several hours before the procedure
- Parenteral fluid replacement (75 ml/hr)
- Three-lead ECG monitoring
- Continuous blood pressure monitoring by the least intrusive method
- Baseline tilt 30–45 minutes
- Pharmacologic provocation if necessary (Isuprel preferred) initiated in the supine position at doses sufficient to increase the heart rate 20–30%
- Nurses or technicians experienced in tilt technique may perform the test if the physician is nearby and immediately available
- Positive test defined as hypotension or bradycardia (or both) with or without reproduction of the patient's symptoms

### Chart 8-6
NEUROCARDIOGENIC PATIENT EDUCATION AND COUNSELING

- Review the pathophysiology of neurocardiogenic syncope
- Address driving restrictions and home and work restrictions as recommended by the physician; refer to state Bureau of Motor Vehicle laws
- Instruct to sit or lie down in the presence of prodromal symptoms
- Instruct to avoid high risk activities if patient has not had prodrome with syncopal spells
- Avoid volume depletion; drink plenty of water and do not restrict salt
- Situational avoidance: avoid any known situation, if possible, that predisposes an individual to neurocardiogenic syncope, such as heat, alcohol, prolonged standing or sitting, pain, large meals, lack of sleep

tonia. Disopyramide (Norpace), which exhibits both negative inotropic actions and anticholinergic effects, has proved helpful in controlling episodes of neurocardiogenic syncope. Theophylline is thought to be effective by blocking the peripheral vasodilatory effects of adenosine. Serotonin reuptake inhibitors, such as sertraline (Zoloft) serve to down-regulate serotonin receptors, which decreases the amount of serotonin surge with stimulation of the medulla vasodepressor center. Because bradycardia is only rarely the proximate cause of neurocardiogenic syncope, pacemakers are generally not helpful. Should a pacemaker be indicated, a dual-chamber device provides the greatest benefit. Commonly used therapies to manage neurocardiogenic syncope are listed in Table 8–2.

## CARDIAC ARRHYTHMIAS CAUSING SYNCOPE

Several diagnostic tests are used to help determine if a cardiac arrhythmia is the cause of syncope. Noninvasive tests include exercise treadmill testing and ambulatory monitoring. Exercise treadmill testing may be helpful for evaluating exercise-induced arrhythmias. Holter monitoring has low diagnostic efficacy for determining the cause of syncope but may be helpful for evaluating patients with passing-out episodes. The use of loop recorders has improved the diagnostic yield of ambulatory monitoring as they may be kept on the patient for up to 1 month. The electrophysiology study is an invasive procedure utilized to evaluate cardiac arrhythmias that contribute to syncope. These arrhythmias are discussed here briefly; more detailed information is provided in Chapters 4 through 7.

| Table 8-2 | COMMONLY USED THERAPIES FOR MANAGEMENT OF NEUROCARDIOGENIC SYNCOPE |
|---|---|
| **THERAPY** | **DOSE (MG/DAY)** |
| β-blockers | |
|   Atenolol | 25–100 |
|   Metoprolol | 25–200 |
|   Propranolol | 40–160 |
| Volume-expanding agents | |
|   Fludrocortisone | 0.1–1.0 |
| Vagolytic agents | |
|   Disopyramide (Norpace) | 200–600 |
| Adenosine antagonists | |
|   Theophylline | 6–12 mg/kg/day |
| Serotonin reuptake inhibitors | |
|   Sertraline (Zoloft) | 50–100 |

Bradycardia is thought to be a common cause of syncope but actually accounts for less than 5% of syncopal episodes. Sinus node dysfunction and AV block are the most common causes of bradycardia.

Supraventricular or ventricular tachycardias may cause syncope. Supraventricular tachycardias are rarely the cause of syncope and are usually associated with other conditions. Atrial fibrillation in patients with Wolff-Parkinson-White syndrome and supraventricular tachycardia triggering neurocardiogenic syncope are two such conditions.

Ventricular tachycardias are the most common cause of syncope in patients with underlying heart disease. Syncopal events due to ventricular arrhythmias usually occur suddenly and without warning and may be preceded by a racing heart sensation. As mentioned previously, syncope in the setting of cardiovascular disease is associated with a high mortality rate and should be evaluated and managed aggressively, as malignant ventricular arrhythmias are often the cause of syncope in these patients.

Approximately 350,000 people per year experience sudden cardiac death in the United States, accounting for nearly 50% of all cardiac deaths. The electrophysiologist is often asked to evaluate patients who have survived an aborted episode of sudden death. This chapter addresses the evaluation of a typical patient surviving an episode of aborted sudden death and the electrophysiologist's role in identifying patients at high risk for sudden cardiac death prior to such an event.

## EVALUATING THE SUDDEN DEATH SURVIVOR

Most patients suffering an episode of aborted sudden cardiac death have underlying coronary artery disease, with an acute myocardial infarction being the primary cause of the cardiac arrest. In patients with myocardial enzyme levels diagnostic of an acute myocardial infarction, the cause of the cardiac arrest is usually presumed to be acute ischemia. Treatment of their coronary ischemia is the primary focus of therapy, and electrophysiologic (EP) testing is not usually necessary. If the patient has a small or insignificant rise in myocardial enzymes, the cause of sudden death is less certain. A study looking for myocardial ischemia is usually performed to evaluate the possibility of underlying significant coronary disease. An assessment of ventricular function [e.g., echocardiogram, multiple gated acquisition (MUGA) blood pool scan] is also usually performed. The probability of inducing ventricular tachycardia at EP testing is significantly increased in patients with coronary artery disease and poor left ventricular function. Possible arrhythmic causes of sudden death that must be considered and evaluated include (1) malignant ventricular arrhythmias; (2) malignant bradyarrhythmias; (3) paroxysmal supraventricular tachycardia (including Wolff-Parkinson-White syndrome); and (4) long QT syndrome/torsade de pointes.

*Malignant ventricular arrhythmias* are diagnosed by electrocardiographic (ECG) monitoring (Holter, event monitors, in-hospital monitors) and by using programmed electrical stimulation of the ventricle (as described in Chapter 7). The sensitivity of programmed ventricular stimulation for sustained ventricular tachycardia is approximately 95% in patients with coronary artery disease and myocardial scarring. If the patient has reproducibly inducible ventricular tachycardia, undergoes antiarrhythmic drug loading, and is found to have no inducible ventricular tachycardia during follow-up EP testing, the 2-year risk of sudden death is decreased to approximately 15%, which compares to a 2-year risk of sudden death of approximately 50% if the ventricular tachycardia is still inducible or no therapy is provided.

Treatment with an implantable defibrillator decreases the risk of sudden death in this group to approximately 2%. In patients with nonischemic dilated cardiomyopathies, programmed stimulation is not as good a predictor of subsequent events. Thus there is an increasing trend toward the use of implantable defibrillators instead of antiarrhythmic therapy in this group of patients.

*Malignant bradyarrhythmias* are a less common cause of cardiac arrest. This possibility can also be evaluated using ECG monitoring (Holter monitors, in-hospital monitoring, or event monitors) in conjunction with EP testing. The EP study is used to evaluate the patient's sinus node function and atrioventricular (AV) conduction (as presented in Chapters 4 and 5) to exclude sinus arrest or intermittent high grade AV conduction block as the cause. Although the specificity of the EP study for these problems is good, the sensitivity is only approximately 70%. Generally, intensive ECG monitoring or empiric pacemaker implantation is undertaken if severe bradyarrhythmias are strongly suspected and the EP study is unrevealing.

Rarely, *paroxysmal supraventricular tachycardia and the Wolff-Parkinson-White (WPW) syndrome* provoke atrial arrhythmias that degenerate into ventricular tachycardia or fibrillation (Figure 9–1). The EP study is extremely sensitive for detecting the presence of these supraventricular arrhythmias and identifying accessory pathway conduction (as described in Chapter 6). Radiofrequency ablation (as described in Chapter 10) is usually the therapy of choice for these patients.

*Long QT syndrome and torsades de pointes* (congenital and acquired) are usually identified by the morphology of the ventricular tachycardia and 12-lead ECG criteria. Treadmill testing, echocardiography, physical signs, and family history as outlined later in this chapter can also be helpful. EP testing is not generally helpful except in rare cases. Therapy of the congenital form of the disease usually involves treatment with some combination of β-blockers, pacing therapy, sympathetic ganglionectomy, and an implantable defibrillator. The acquired form is usually treated by addressing the underlying cause (e.g., electrolyte imbalance, pharmacologic agents).

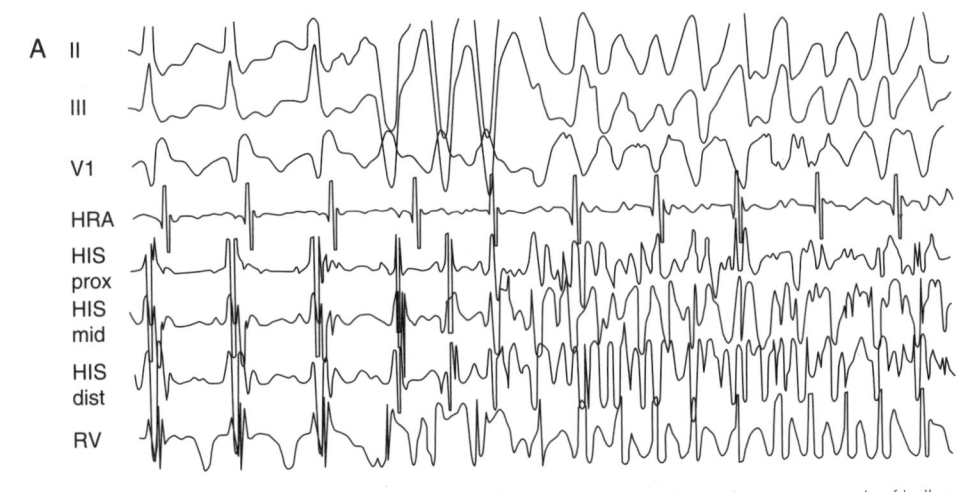

**Figure 9-1 • (A)** Degeneration of typical paroxysmal supraventricular tachycardia into ventricular fibrillation. The intracardiac electrograms confirm that the inciting arrhythmia is AV node reentrant tachycardia. *Illustration continued on opposite page.*

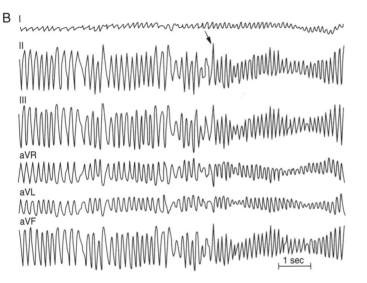

**Figure 9-1 • *Continued***
**(B)** Atrial fibrillation conducting over an accessory pathway degenerating into ventricular fibrillation. Arrow marks the onset of ventricular fibrillation.

159

## IDENTIFYING PATIENTS AT RISK FOR SUDDEN DEATH

The electrophysiologist not only manages patients who present with aborted episodes of sudden death but also attempts to identify patients at particularly high risk for a future malignant arrhythmic event so as to take preventive action. In the remainder of this chapter we classify patients at high risk for a sudden arrhythmic event by their underlying substrate and discuss the methods of risk stratification and types of therapy available.

### Coronary Artery Disease

Autopsy reports indicate that 80% of patients experiencing sudden cardiac death suffer from severe coronary artery disease. One of five myocardial infarctions first present as sudden cardiac death. In patients with coronary artery disease who do not have acutely infarcting myocardium, the most common cause of sudden death is ventricular tachycardia that degenerates into ventricular fibrillation. A reentrant circuit utilizing scar tissue is thought to be the most common mechanism. Certain factors have been found to be indicative of an increased risk of sudden death in patients with coronary artery disease:

1. Left ventricular ejection fraction <40%
2. Late potentials on signal average ECG
3. Decreased heart rate variability
4. Nonsustained ventricular tachycardia
5. History of syncope

Programmed stimulation of the ventricle is both sensitive and specific for further delineating the risk in this population. If a patient with an ejection fraction of <40% is found to have no inducible ventricular tachycardia during programmed stimulation, the risk of sudden death is approximately 5% per year; a positive study confers a 35–45% risk, often indicating the need for intervention with drug or device therapy.

## Idiopathic Dilated Cardiomyopathy

Survival of patients with idiopathic dilated cardiomyopathy is approximately 70% at 1 year and 50% at 2 years after presentation. Approximately 30–70% of deaths in this group of patients are sudden. The primary cause of sudden death in these patients is thought to be secondary to ventricular tachycardia/fibrillation, but there also may be a significant role for bradyarrhythmic death. Assessment of risk in these patients is controversial, yet certain factors predict an increased future risk of sudden death:

1. History of aborted sudden death
2. Nonsustained ventricular tachycardia
3. History of syncope

In these patients the absence of inducible monomorphic ventricular tachycardia during programmed stimulation does not confer a significantly lower risk of sudden death; however, induction of monomorphic ventricular tachycardia predicts a markedly increased future risk for sudden death. Therapy in these patients currently consists of empiric amiodarone for asymptomatic high risk patients and implantable defibrillator implantation for symptomatic high risk patients. There is also a trend toward increased use of implantable defibrillators in some asymptomatic patients.

## Hypertrophic Cardiomyopathy

The prevalence of hypertrophic cardiomyopathy, a genetic disorder of myocardial hypertrophy—commonly referred to as idiopathic hypertrophic subaortic stenosis (IHSS) or hypertrophic obstructive cardiomyopathy (HOCM)—is approximately 20 per 100,000 in the U.S. population. Although this disorder has a mortality of approximately 2% per year, most of these deaths are sudden in a generally young population. Most of the deaths are thought to be due to ventricular arrhythmias caused by abnormal calcium ion regulation, nonuniform distribution of action potential duration, and abnormal passive electrical propagation in the ventricular myocardium. Sudden death appears to be more common in the patients with the following criteria:

1. Age less than 30 years
2. Family history of sudden death
3. Nonsustained ventricular tachycardia

The lack of understanding of the underlying cause of arrhythmia in these patients and the marginal applicability of programmed stimulation of the ventricle for risk stratification makes their management difficult. Currently, most survivors of sudden death or patients with symptomatic ventricular tachycardia receive implantable defibrillators.

## Idiopathic and Acquired Long QT Syndrome

Idiopathic long QT syndrome is genetically linked with fewer than 10% of cases being reported as sporadic. The Jervell and Lange-Nielsen form of the disease is marked by:

1. Congenital deafness
2. Recurrent syncope or sudden death
3. Family history of sudden death (recessive pattern)
4. QT prolongation

The Romano-Ward form of the disease is marked by:

1. Syncope and sudden death
2. Family history of sudden death (dominant pattern)
3. QT prolongation

A QTc of more than 0.44 seconds has been the accepted criterion for QT prolongation, but it is now adjusted for age and sex. Other ECG findings, such as bifid T waves and marked sinus bradycardia, help strengthen clinical suspicion and diagnosis. Evaluation includes Holter monitoring, treadmill testing, and in some cases echocardiographic contraction patterns. Documenting torsades de pointes on ECG monitoring confirms the diagnosis. EP testing is not generally useful, except when monophasic action potentials are used to record after-depolarizations. Therapy usually consists of some combination of β-blocker treatment, pacemaker placement, left cervicothoracic sympathetic ganglionectomy, or implantable defibrillator implantation. Acquired long QT syndrome is marked by a long QT interval that is exacerbated during the pause-dependent onset of torsades de pointes (Figure 9–2). The acquired form of long QT syndrome is usually caused by:

1. Pharmacologic agents (e.g., antiarrhythmics, phenothiazines, tricyclic antidepressants)
2. Electrolyte disorders (hypokalemia, hypomagnesemia)
3. Bradyarrhythmias
4. Miscellaneous substances (e.g., liquid protein diet)

The cause is usually readily apparent after the differential diagnosis is investigated. Treatment involves removing the offending agent or correcting the underlying abnormality. Temporizing measures include catecholamine infusion, intravenous magnesium, or overdrive pacing.

## Arrhythmogenic Right Ventricular Dysplasia

Arrhythmogenic right ventricular dysplasia (ARVD) is one of the few causes of sudden cardiac death in young, healthy people who have no overt evidence of cardiac disease. ARVD is caused by fatty replacement of the right ventricular myocardium and may be the result of previously healed myocarditis. Life-threatening arrhythmias appear to be the most prominent manifestation of this disease, often occurring during exercise. The overall risk of death is 2% per year despite treatment. Diagnosis of this disorder requires

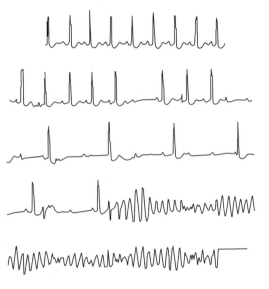

**Figure 9-2** • Typical pause-dependent QT prolongation with onset of torsade de pointes (polymorphic ventricular tachycardia) in a patient with acquired long QT syndrome due to intermittent complete heart block.

a high level of suspicion, as there is often no significant right ventricular disease noted on routine surface echocardiography. The diagnosis is usually established by the presence of a right ventricular fatty infiltrate noted on cardiac magnetic resonance imaging or by right ventricular akinesis or dyskinesis noted during right ventriculography. These patients also have markedly abnormal signal-averaged ECGs with delayed potentials extending beyond the limit of the window. Certain surface ECG criteria can also indicate the presence of this disorder. Appropriate therapy for this disorder is primarily focused on eliminating or decreasing the risk of sudden cardiac death. Pharmacologic options are almost entirely limited to amiodarone or sotalol. There has been a lower threshold for using implantable defibrillators in this group of patients.

## Wolff-Parkinson-White Syndrome

The WPW syndrome is rare but can cause sudden cardiac death in an otherwise perfectly healthy patient. The prevalence of WPW syndrome in the population is approximately 0.3% with an attendant risk of sudden death of anywhere from 0.5% to 4.0%. The mechanism of sudden death is thought to be secondary to unrestricted antegrade conduction of atrial fibrillation to the ventricle over an accessory pathway with subsequent induction of ventricular fibrillation (Figure 9–3). Risk stratification of these patients is based on profiles of patients with WPW syndrome who were resuscitated from sudden cardiac death. Ninety percent of resuscitated patients had minor to significantly symptomatic arrhythmias; the other 10% were entirely asymptomatic. Thus although a lack of symptoms does not free one from risk, the presence of symptoms is certainly cause for concern. With few exceptions, patients who suffer a cardiac arrest manifest the abil-

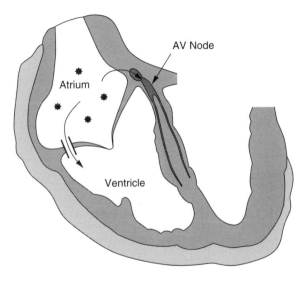

**Figure 9-3** • Route of unrestrained conduction of atrial fibrillation over an accessory pathway, in contrast to slower conduction over the atrioventricular (AV) node.

ity to conduct rapidly over their accessory pathway with the shortest RR interval between preexcited beats being less than 250 ms.

At this point, any patient with WPW syndrome and symptomatic tachycardia would be advised to undergo an EP evaluation and possibly radiofrequency ablation of the accessory pathway. Asymptomatic patients can probably be followed clinically until they become symptomatic. Exceptions are asymptomatic WPW patients in whom rapid conduction over the accessory pathway is noted during an EP study, patients in whom even the possibility of an arrhythmia is unacceptable (e.g., airline pilots, armed forces personnel), and those who cannot emotionally tolerate their condition.

# CHAPTER 10

# RADIOFREQUENCY CATHETER ABLATION

Over the last decade, radiofrequency ablation techniques have revolutionized the treatment of many arrhythmias. Both supraventricular and ventricular arrhythmias are amenable to treatment with catheter ablation; and for some arrhythmias it is now considered the primary therapy. This chapter describes the indications, mapping techniques, methods of radiofrequency application, and endpoints for successful ablation for various arrhythmias treatable with this technology.

## COMPLETE ATRIOVENTRICULAR JUNCTION ABLATION

### Indications

The major indications for ablating the atrioventricular (AV) junction are for rate or symptom control in patients with chronic or paroxysmal atrial fibrillation refractory to medical management. This type of therapy is palliative, not curative, in these patients because the atrial fibrillation is still present. They continue to require long-term warfarin (Coumadin) therapy if they can tolerate anticoagulation. After ablation of the AV junction and creation of complete heart block, pacemaker therapy is required. In patients with paroxysmal atrial fibrillation, a dual-chamber pacemaker with automatic mode switching capabilities can often be utilized to maintain normal AV synchrony. In patients with chronic atrial fibrillation, a ventricular rate-responsive pacemaker is the preferred pacing modality. Approximately 85% of patients with medically refractory rapid atrial fibrillation show symptomatic improvement after AV junction ablation.

## Mapping

The AV junction can be ablated using a right- or left-side approach (Figure 10–1). With the right-side approach the catheter is positioned along the tricuspid annulus close to the standard His bundle recording position. With the left-side approach the catheter is positioned across the aortic valve at the summit of the left ventricular septum. In general, the right-side approach is tried first and is effective in more than 85% of cases. The left-side approach is usually reserved for patients in whom the right-side approach fails. For a right-side ablation the catheter is positioned so sizable atrial, His bundle, and ventricular electrograms are simultaneously recorded (Figure 10–2). The most common mistake is to position the catheter tip too far distally along the His-Purkinje axis so only the right bundle branch is ablated when the radiofrequency current is applied. This distal positioning is indicated by seeing only a small or nonexistent atrial electrogram at a position where large His bundle and ventricular electrograms are seen. For a left-side ablation the catheter is positioned across the aortic valve, and the summit of the left ventricular septum is mapped to find a large His bundle electrogram. Unlike the right-side approach, the atrial electrograms at successful sites on the left side are often small (Figure 10–3).

## Radiofrequency Application and Determinants of Success

After a site has been selected, radiofrequency current is usually applied at power outputs of 25–35 watts for 30–60 seconds. If temperature guidance is used, temperatures of $60°–70°C$ are needed to ensure adequate heating.

At most successful sites, a junctional rhythm appears within a few seconds of the radiofrequency energy application, and complete heart block often occurs within 10 seconds (Figure 10–4). The endpoint for a successful ablation is the presence of complete heart block. Patients generally have junctional escape rhythms at rates of 30–50 bpm after the ablation procedure.

## Complications

The immediate complications of AV junction ablation are primarily those related to catheter-induced trauma, such as cardiac perforation and tamponade; fortunately, these events are rare. If a left-side approach is used there is also potential for arterial bleeding complications from cannulation of the femoral artery and for complications related to catheter-induced trauma of the aorta, aortic valve, and coronary arteries, along with the risk of thromboembolic events. These complications are also rare and are inherent to any ablation

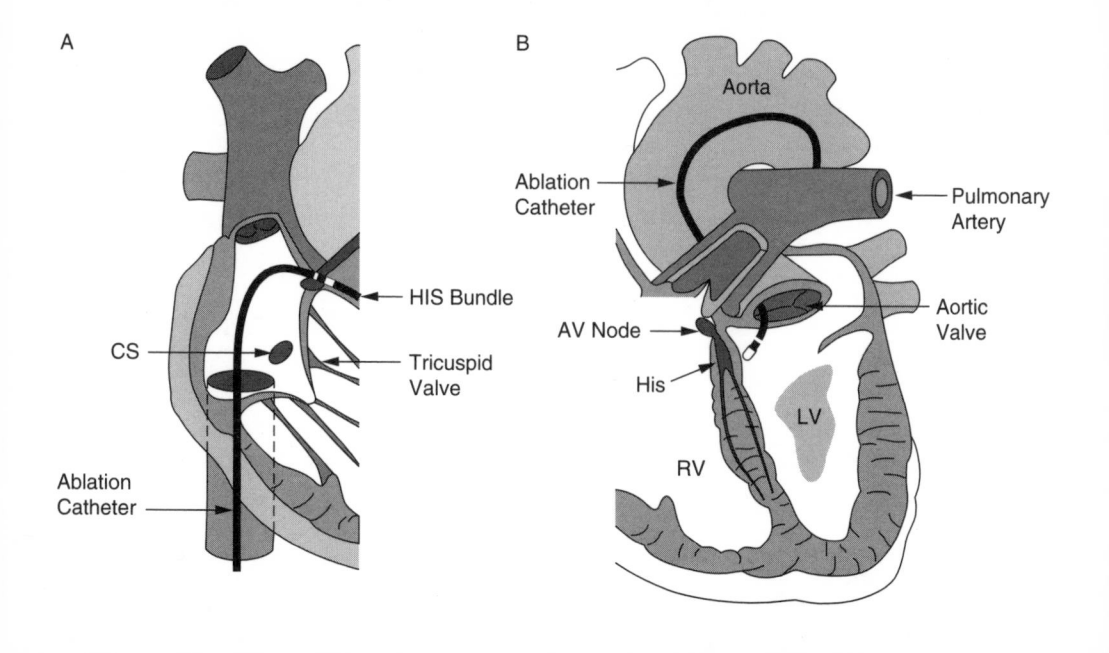

**Figure 10-1** • AV junction ablation: catheter positions for ablation of the AV junction using the right-side **(A)** or left-side **(B)** approach. With the right-side approach, the catheter is positioned along the superior medial aspect of the tricuspid annulus near the typical His bundle recording position. With the left-side approach, the ablation catheter is positioned across the aortic valve along the superior aspect of the left ventricular septum where a His bundle potential is recorded. RV = right ventricle; LV = left ventricle; CS = coronary sinus.

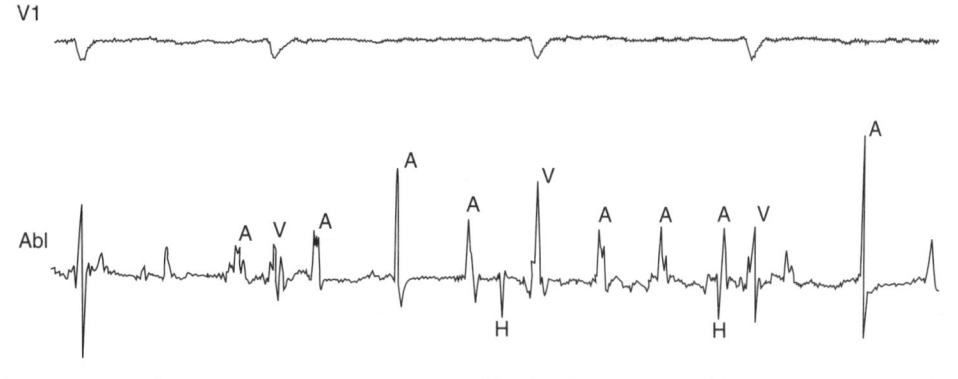

**Figure 10-2 •** Electrogram appearance at a successful right-side AV junction ablation site in a patient who is in atrial fibrillation. Shown is a recording from surface lead $V_1$ and intracardiac recordings from the ablation catheter (Abl) positioned proximally in the His bundle region. Note that the atrial electrograms (A) are as large as or larger than the ventricular electrograms (V) and that there is also a large His bundle deflection (H). The A/V electrogram ratio of ≥1.0 indicates that this site is proximal in the His bundle region.

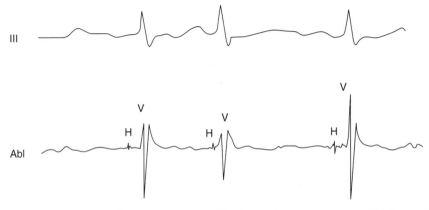

**Figure 10-3** • These tracings, from a patient in atrial fibrillation, demonstrate a successful left-side AV junction ablation site. Shown are a recording from surface lead III and intracardiac recordings from the ablation catheter (Abl). The recordings on the ablation catheter demonstrate a large ventricular electrogram (V) and sizable His bundle deflections (H) but essentially no atrial activity.

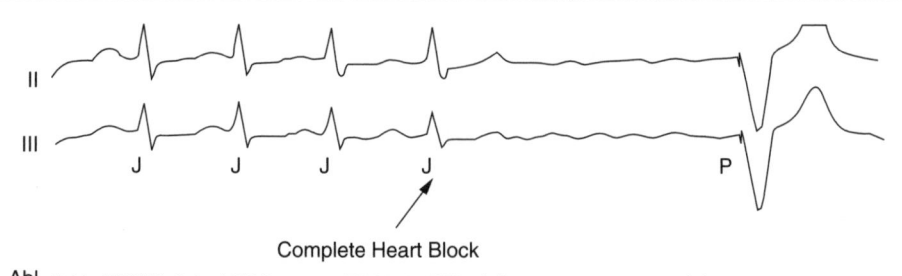

**Figure 10–4** • AV junction ablation. These tracings show the effect of radiofrequency (RF) current application at a successful AV junction ablation site. Shown are recordings from surface leads II and III, and from the ablation catheter (Abl). With the RF current turned on, the ablation catheter does not record any electrical activity. During RF application the patient developed an accelerated junctional rhythm (J), and complete heart block was created after 6 seconds of current application. The patient had a ventricular pacemaker placed prior to the ablation procedure setup at a backup rate of 40 bpm. Ventricular pacing (P) ensued upon creation of complete AV block.

that uses a left-side retrograde aortic approach. After AV junction ablation small numbers of patients have developed polymorphic ventricular tachycardia, which can be life-threatening. It appears to be a rate-related phenomenon and can usually be avoided by pacing patients at rates of 80 bpm or more for at least 24 hours after the procedure.

## AV NODE MODIFICATION

### Indications

Atrioventricular node modification is used for treating patients with AV node reentrant tachycardia (AVNRT). The primary indication for ablation is to treat patients with recurrent tachycardias who are refractory or intolerant of medical therapy. Today radiofrequency ablation is frequently being used as primary therapy for treating PSVT. This approach should be strongly considered in patients with significant symptoms such as syncope associated with their tachycardia. The success rate of AV node modification for treating AVNRT is better than 95%, with complication rates of less than 1% at experienced centers.

### Mapping

Patients with typical AVNRT have both a fast and a slow AV nodal pathway. AV node modification can be performed by selectively ablating either of these pathways (Figure 10–5). The fast pathway is located in close proximity to the compact AV node, just slightly proximal to the normal His bundle recording posi-

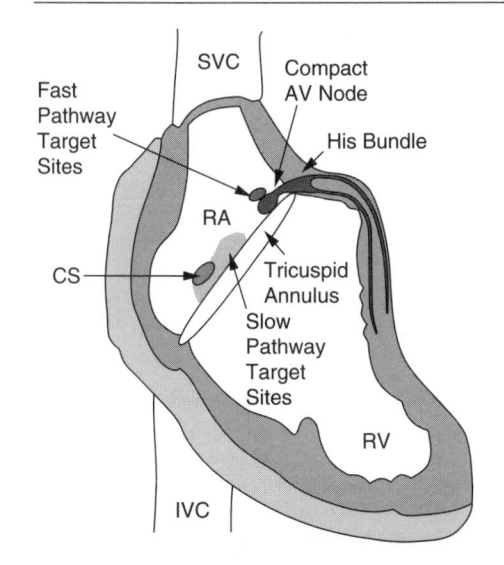

**Figure 10-5 •** Usual target locations for the fast and slow pathways involved in AV node reentrant tachycardia. The fast pathway is usually located anteriorly just proximal to the compact AV node. The slow pathway is usually located more posteriorly along the tricuspid annulus near the coronary sinus (CS) ostium. RA = right atrium; SVC = superior vena cava; IVC = inferior vena cava; RV = right ventricle.

tion. The fast pathway approach, which was the first to be used, was associated with a relatively high incidence of complete heart block. This fact has led to the abandonment of this approach in favor of the slow pathway technique. The slow AV nodal pathway is located posterior to the compact AV node, usually near the coronary sinus ostium.

A common technique for localizing the slow pathway is to use a combined anatomic and atrial electrogram mapping approach. The ablation catheter is positioned along the tricuspid annulus inferior to the His bundle recording area near the coronary sinus ostium. This region is mapped looking for fractionated atrial electrograms with an atrial/ventricular electrogram ratio of 0.5 or less (Figure 10–6). If no acceptable electrograms are found, a purely anatomic approach can be used. With this approach, radiofrequency lesions are delivered in a systematic fashion along the tricuspid annulus near the coronary sinus ostium. The lesions are usually created progressing from inferior to superior locations to minimize the risk of applying the radiofrequency current close to the AV node. The electrograms recorded from each potential ablation site should be scrutinized closely to evaluate for a His bundle potential. If a His bundle potential is recorded, an alternative site is usually sought to minimize the risk of creating complete heart block.

## Radiofrequency Application

Once an acceptable location is found, radiofrequency (RF) energy is delivered, usually with power outputs of 25–40 watts. During energy application, the rhythm is monitored closely to detect signs of AV block. At successful slow pathway sites, a junctional rhythm usually emerges during the RF application. With this

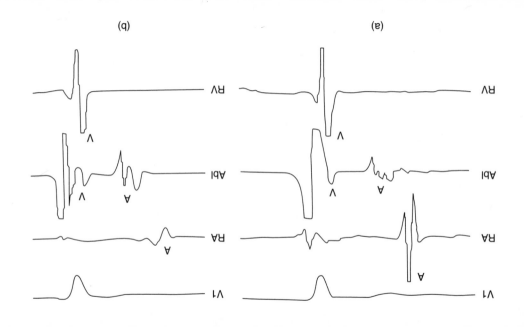

**Figure 10-6 •** Slow pathway ablation sites. **(a, b)** Recording from surface lead $V_1$ and intracardiac recordings from the right atrium (RA), ablation catheter (Abl), and right ventricle (RV) are shown. The ablation catheter is positioned along the tricuspid annulus near the coronary sinus. Both recordings are typical of successful slow pathway ablation sites. Note the fractionated atrial electrogram (A) and A/V electrogram ratio of ≤0.5 on the ablation catheter recording. V = Ventricular electrogram.

junctional rhythm, there is usually 1:1 retrograde VA conduction, presumably via the fast pathway (Figure 10–7). The retrograde conduction is monitored closely; and if VA block is seen, the RF application should be terminated immediately. The occurrence of VA block during junctional rhythm is a predictor of complete heart block. At locations remote from the AV node, the RF energy can be applied safely at higher power outputs. At locations closer to the AV node, a safer approach is to titrate the energy application usually starting at power outputs of 10–15 watts and titrating upward to energies of 25–40 watts while monitoring for the emergence of a junctional rhythm or the occurrence of AV block. For AV node modification, temperature monitoring has not been found to offer a significant advantage over impedance monitoring presumably because the occurrence of a junctional rhythm during the application ensures that adequate heating is taking place.

## Determinants of Success

The most important endpoint for successful AV node modification, as with all ablations, is the elimination of inducible tachycardia. In all patients with AVNRT retesting must be performed in the baseline state and with AV nodal-enhancing drugs such as isoproterenol. In some cases the tachycardia may have been difficult to reproducibly initiate. Therefore a lack of inducibility after RF applications does not always guarantee long-term success. In these cases other secondary endpoints may be used. The optimal endpoint of a slow pathway ablation is complete elimination of slow pathway function, which is usually demonstrated by showing the lack of an AV nodal jump when one was present before the ablation (Figure 10–8). In most

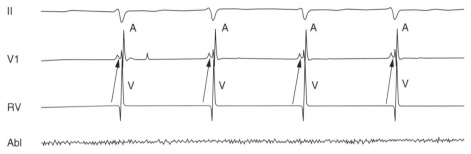

**Figure 10-7** • Junctional rhythm with radiofrequency (RF) application. These recordings were made during radiofrequency (RF) current application at a successful slow pathway ablation site. Shown are a recording from surface lead V₁ and intracardiac recordings from the right atrium (RA), right ventricle (RV), and ablation catheter (Abl). No intracardiac electrograms are seen on the ablation catheter during the RF current application. All four beats shown are junctional beats that emerged during the RF application. Note that with each junctional beat seen on the RV tracing (V) there is a corresponding atrial electrogram (A) on the right atrial tracings, presumably because of retrograde conduction from the junction to the atrium via the fast pathway. This pattern of conduction must be monitored closely; and if VA block is seen, the RF application should be terminated immediately because of the risk of creating complete AV block.

A

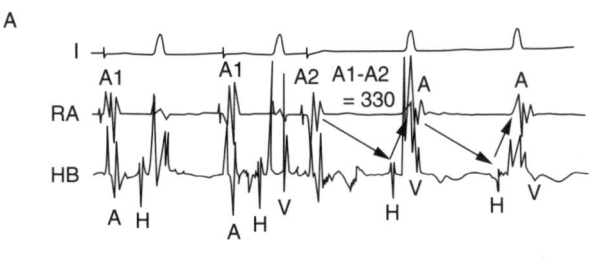

B

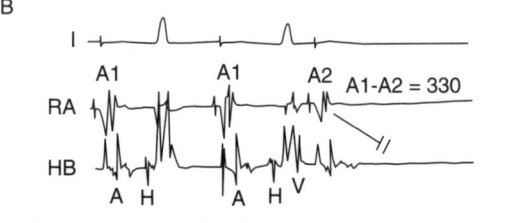

**Figure 10-8** • Elimination of slow pathway function. **(A, B)** Shown are recordings from surface lead I and intracardiac recordings from the right atrium (RA) and His bundle region (HB). **(A)** Recorded prior to the slow pathway ablation. The right atrium was paced using an eight-beat drive train (A1–A1 = 500 ms), and a premature stimulus (A2) was delivered at a coupling interval of 330 ms. With this pacing scheme, A2 conducted via the slow pathway and tachycardia was induced. **(B)** Recorded after ablation of the slow pathway. The same pacing scheme as in **A** was used, but this time the premature beat A2 was blocked because the slow pathway has been eliminated.

cases ablation of the slow pathway is also associated with an increase in the AV block cycle length and the inability to create long AH intervals during atrial overdrive pacing. In some patients complete elimination of slow pathway function is not necessary, and attenuation of slow pathway function is acceptable. In these cases, an AV nodal jump and single AV nodal echoes may persist, but the ability of the slow pathway to sustain tachycardia is gone. If more than a single AV nodal echo is present, continued RF ablation attempts are generally required.

## Complications

The major complication of AV node modification is creation of complete heart block. Using the slow pathway approach, this problem is rare, occurring in fewer than 1% of cases at experienced centers. Other potential complications are those related to vascular or myocardial trauma inherent in any invasive electrophysiology procedure.

## ACCESSORY PATHWAY ABLATION

### Indications

As with AV node modification, the primary indication for accessory pathway ablation is to treat recurrent medically refractory tachycardias. More frequently it is being used as primary therapy especially in patients who present with serious arrhythmias associated with the Wolff-Parkinson-White (WPW) syndrome. One of the most significant arrhythmias in this patient group is atrial fibrillation with a rapid ventricular response resulting from conduction across the accessory pathway (Figure 10–9). It leads to an irregular wide complex tachycardia that can have rates of 300 bpm or more and in some cases results in cardiovascular collapse and sudden death. The success rate for accessory pathways ablation is approximately 95%, and the incidence of serious complications is less than 2%.

## Mapping

Overt accessory pathways can be mapped using antegrade or retrograde conduction timing parameters, whereas concealed accessory pathways can be mapped using only retrograde timing parameters. Mapping using antegrade conduction is usually performed with the patient in normal sinus rhythm. In some cases atrial overdrive pacing may be used to accentuate the degree of ventricular preexcitation. With this mapping approach, a location along the tricuspid annulus (for right-side accessory pathways) or the mitral annulus (for left-side accessory pathways) is sought that has the earliest local ventricular electrogram time relative to the onset of the QRS complex. The timing of the local ventricular electrogram is usually measured at the peak of the major deflection in the electrogram rather than at its onset (Figure 10–10). Sites with ventricular activation times that coincide with the onset of the QRS complex or are before it are generally required for the ablation to be successful.

Mapping using retrograde conduction timing is useful for overt or concealed accessory pathways. With this technique, retrograde conduction across the accessory pathways is established by inducing ortho-

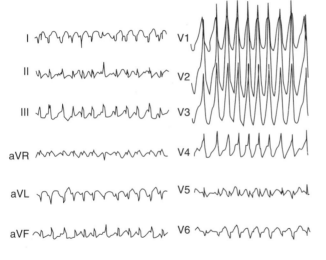

**Figure 10-9 •** Twelve-lead ECG from a patient with Wolff-Parkinson-White syndrome who is in atrial fibrillation. Note the irregular wide complex tachycardia with rates up to 250 bpm. The appearance of the ECG is a result of the atrial fibrillation impulses conducting across the accessory pathway to the ventricle.

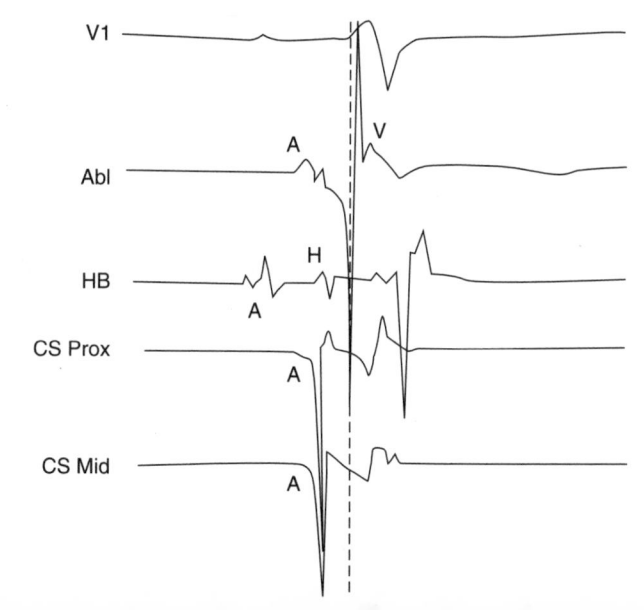

**Figure 10-10** • Overt accessory pathway ablation site: recording from surface lead $V_1$ and intracardiac recordings from the ablation catheter (Abl) located along the lateral mitral annulus, His bundle recording position (HB), and proximal and mid coronary sinus positions (CS Prox, CS Mid). Note that on the ablation catheter the atrial and ventricular electrograms appear fused and that the peak of the ventricular electrogram appears to coincide with the onset of the QRS complex (dotted line). Local ventricular activation coincident with or before the onset of the QRS complex indicates that this is a good site for radiofrequency application.

dromic reciprocating tachycardia or by ventricular overdrive pacing. Sites along the tricuspid or mitral annulus are sought that have the earliest atrial activation time. During orthodromic reciprocating tachycardia, successful sites often have nearly continuous electrical activity with no isoelectric interval between the local ventricular or atrial electrograms. When mapping during orthodromic reciprocating tachycardia or ventricular pacing, a reliable stable reference point is required from which to measure the atrial timing. Common reference points are the onset of the QRS complex (used during orthodromic tachycardia) and the pacing stimulus (used during ventricular overdrive pacing) (Figure 10–11).

## Radiofrequency Application

After appropriate sites have been selected, the RF current is usually applied at 25–35 watts for 30–60 seconds. At most successful sites accessory pathway function is eliminated less than 5 seconds after the RF current is turned on. If accessory pathway function persists more than 10–15 seconds, the current is shut off to minimize the risk of edema or coagulum formation. A coagulum forms if the catheter tip reaches a temperature of approximately 100°C. For concealed accessory pathways, the RF current is often applied during tachycardia or with ventricular pacing so the efficacy of the application can be monitored. If temperature monitoring is used, temperatures are generally set between 60° and 80°C to ensure adequate heating. Temperature monitoring has the advantage of ensuring that there is adequate heating at a site, and it minimizes the risk of coagulum formation. The latter may be particularly helpful with left-side pathways to decrease the risk of thromboemboli.

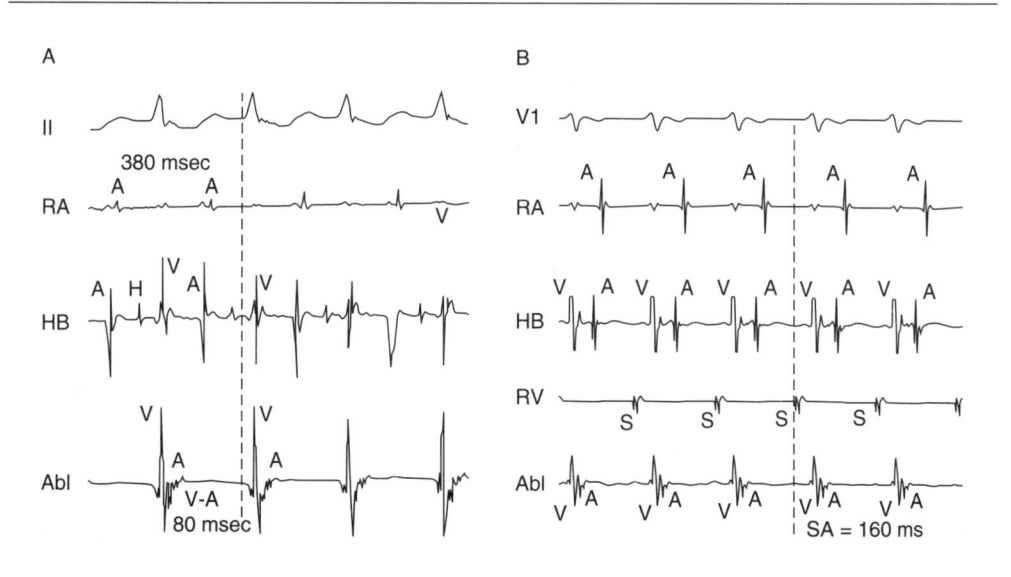

**Figure 10–11 •** Retrograde mapping. **(A)** Recording from surface lead II and intracardiac recordings from the right atrial (RA) and His bundle (HB) regions, and an ablation catheter (Abl). **(B)** Recording from surface lead $V_1$, the right atrium (RA), His bundle region (HB), right ventricle (RV), and ablation catheter (Abl). **(A)** Recordings were made during orthodromic reciprocating tachycardia (ORT). Note that on the ablation catheter (located along the anterolateral mitral annulus) that the ventricular (V) and atrial (A) electrograms are fused. The VA time measured from the onset of the QRS complex to the local atrial electrogram on the ablation catheter was 80 ms, which was the shortest VA time found. This short VA time and electrogram fusion on the ablation catheter during ORT indicate that this is a good ablation site. **(B)** Mapping of a concealed accessory pathway during ventricular pacing. With the ablation catheter positioned along the posterior mitral annulus, a site was found with a pacing stimulus (S)-to-local atrial (A) electrogram time of 160 ms, which was the shortest time found. Radiofrequency application at this site was successful in eliminating accessory pathway function.

## Determinants of Success

For overt accessory pathways, the primary endpoint for success is loss of preexcitation (Figure 10–12A). In most cases loss of antegrade accessory pathway function correlates with loss of retrograde function. For concealed accessory pathways, the primary endpoint is loss of retrograde pathway function (Figure 10–12B), which is confirmed by finding either complete ventriculoatrial disassociation during ventricular pacing (Figure 10–13) or a shift in the atrial activation sequence from eccentric to concentric during ventricular pacing, usually with a significant increase in the ventriculoatrial block cycle length.

## Complications

The most serious complications are related to catheter-induced trauma or the formation of thromboemboli during left-side ablations. These complications include coronary artery dissection with resultant myocardial infarction, aortic and aortic-valve damage, transient ischemic attacks, and cerebral vascular accidents. Fortunately, these events are rare, occurring in fewer than 2% of patients at experienced centers. The risk of aortic, aortic-valve, and coronary artery damage can be minimized by using a transseptal approach rather than a retrograde aortic approach to obtain access to the mitral annulus. This practice, however, exposes the patient to the risks inherent in a transseptal puncture and does not eliminate the risk of thromboembolic complications.

## ATRIAL TACHYCARDIA ABLATION

### Indications

The major indication for ablation of an atrial tachycardia is the same as for the other two forms of paroxysmal supraventricular tachycardia (PSVT), which is recurrent medically refractory tachycardia. The success rate for ablation of atrial tachycardias is on the order of 70–80%, compared to the better than 95% success with AVNRTs and accessory pathway tachycardias.

### Mapping

The primary method for mapping an atrial tachycardia is activation mapping. With this technique, the ablation catheter is moved around the atria during tachycardia, searching for the site of earliest atrial activation (Figure 10–14). For left atrial tachycardias, a transseptal approach via either a patent foramen ovale or transseptal puncture is required to map the left atrium. The activation time recorded from the ablation catheter is measured relative to a stable reference point, which is usually either the onset of the surface P wave or an intracardiac recording from the right atrium. In many cases the onset of the surface of the P wave is difficult to discern, and an intracardiac reference electrogram may be preferred. Successful ablation sites usually have activation times of –20 to –50 ms relative to the onset of the surface P wave.

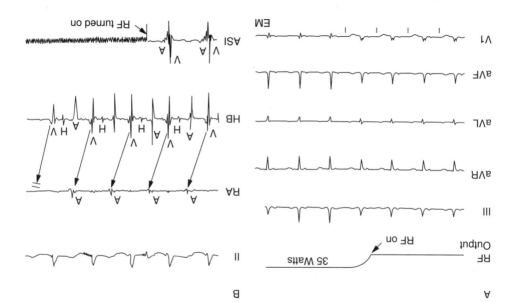

**Figure 10-12 • (A)** Patient with an overt accessory pathway. Radiofrequency (RF) output and recordings from surface leads III, aVR, aVL, aVF, and V$_1$ are shown. Within one beat of the RF current being turned on, the accessory pathway was eliminated. Note the change in the QRS morphology and elimination of the delta wave. **(B)** Tracings are the same as those in Figure 10–11A. The patient was in orthodromic reciprocating tachycardia. When the RF current is turned on, the ablation catheter (Abl) electrograms are lost. Note that on the third beat after the start of the RF application retrograde conduction to the atrium is blocked because of elimination of accessory pathway function.

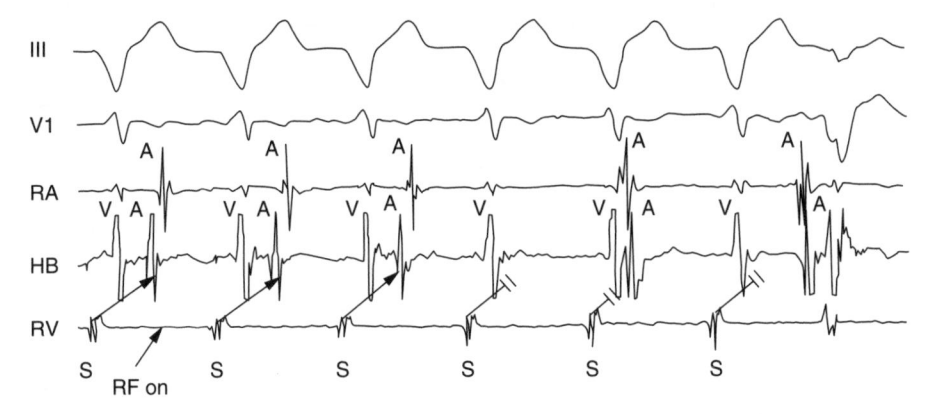

**Figure 10–13 •** Recordings from surface leads III and V$_1$ and intracardiac recordings from the right atrium (RA), His bundle region (HB), and right ventricle (RV). The patient was being ventricularly paced (S) at a cycle length of 500 ms. The ablation catheter (not shown) was positioned along the posterior mitral annulus. The radiofrequency (RF) current application was started after the first paced beat as indicated. Note that with the first three paced beats there is 1:1 ventriculoatrial (VA) conduction. On the fourth paced beat VA conduction is lost, indicating successful ablation of the accessory pathway.

## Radiofrequency Ablation

Once an appropriate site is selected, RF current is usually applied at power outputs of 20–35 watts or temperature settings of 60°–80°C for 30–60 seconds.

## Determinants of Success

Initial success is indicated by termination of the tachycardia during the RF application (Figure 10–15), which usually occurs within seconds of turning on the RF current at an appropriate site. The only good predictor of long-term success is the inability to reinduce the tachycardia after its termination.

## Complications

The most common complications during atrial tachycardia ablations are those related to catheter-induced trauma. Thromboembolic events with a transseptal approach for left atrial ablations are also possible. Complications are fortunately rare when appropriate precautions are taken.

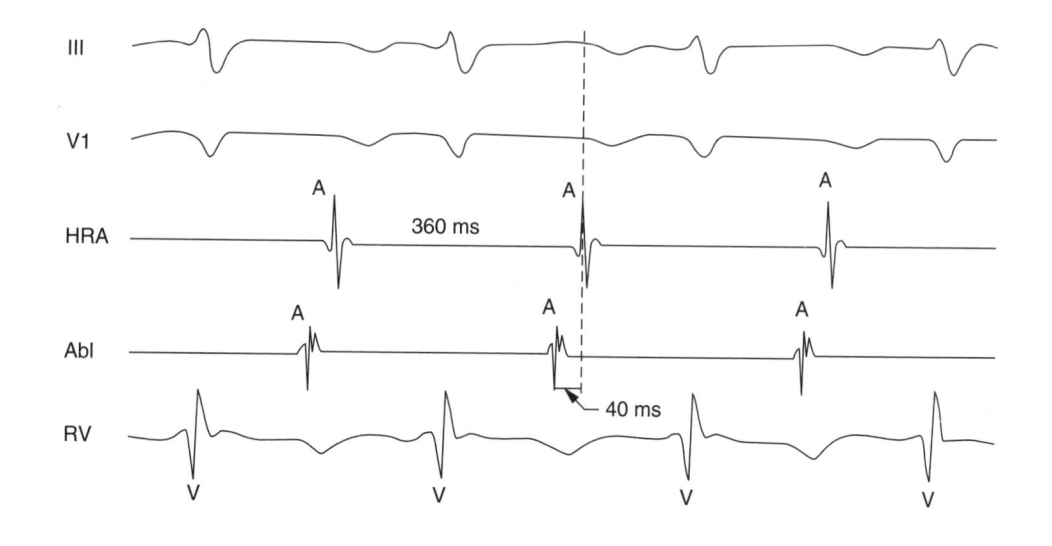

**Figure 10-14** • Atrial tachycardia activation mapping. Shown are recordings from surface leads III and V₁ and intracardiac recordings from the high right atrium (HRA), ablation catheter (Abl), and right ventricle (RV). The patient was in atrial tachycardia at a cycle length of 360 ms. The ablation catheter was positioned along the lateral aspect of the right atrium. The activation time was measured relative to the onset of the high right atrial catheter, which coincided with the onset of the surface P wave. At this site, the activation time was 40 ms prior to the onset of the atrial electrogram in the high right atrium. Radiofrequency current application at this site resulted in successful ablation of the atrial tachycardia.

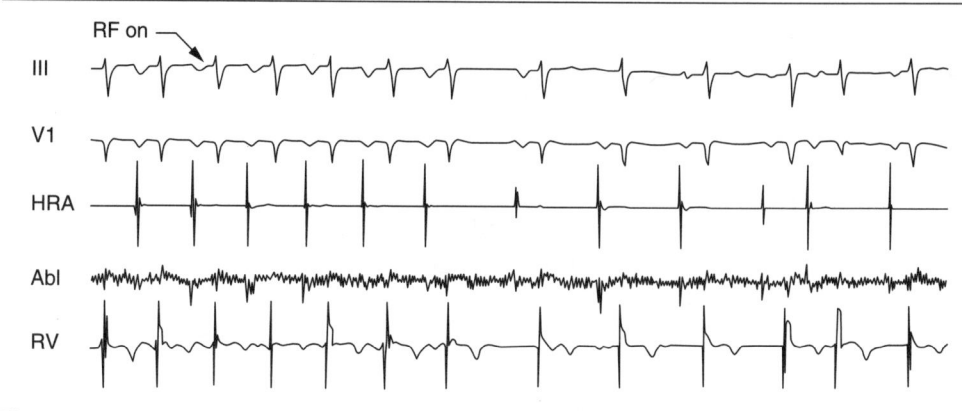

**Figure 10–15 •** Termination of atrial tachycardia with radiofrequency (RF) application. Shown are recordings from surface leads III and $V_1$ and intracardiac recordings from the high right atrium (HRA), ablation catheter (Abl), and right ventricle (RV). The ablation catheter was located along the lateral aspect of the right atrium as shown in Figure 10–14. Note that with the ablation application no intracardiac electrograms are recorded on the ablation catheter. After the RF energy was turned on, the tachycardia terminated within four beats and sinus rhythm was restored.

## ATRIAL FLUTTER

### Indications

Patients best suited for ablation therapy of atrial flutter are those with recurrent or chronic typical atrial flutter (Figure 10–16) without other associated atrial arrhythmias. The primary success rate for ablation of typical atrial flutter is approximately 90% with recurrence rates of approximately 10–15%. Patients with a history of atrial fibrillation have a high incidence of recurrent atrial fibrillation after cure of their atrial flutter and therefore are probably best treated with drug therapy if they are appropriate candidates. In some of these patients drug therapy suppresses the atrial fibrillation but not the atrial flutter. In these cases a stepwise approach of drug therapy followed by catheter ablation may be useful.

### Mapping

The approach for ablation of atrial flutter is primarily anatomic. The isthmus of atrial tissue between the inferior vena cava and tricuspid valve is a critical portion of the atrial flutter circuit (Figure 10–17). The usual ablation technique is to create a line of block in this region by applying sequential RF lesions between the tricuspid valve and the inferior vena cava. The location of the ablation tip is determined using a combination of fluoroscopy and electrogram analysis (Figure 10–18). The more distal locations along the isthmus are close to the tricuspid valve and have a small atrial/ventricular electrogram ratio. As the abla-

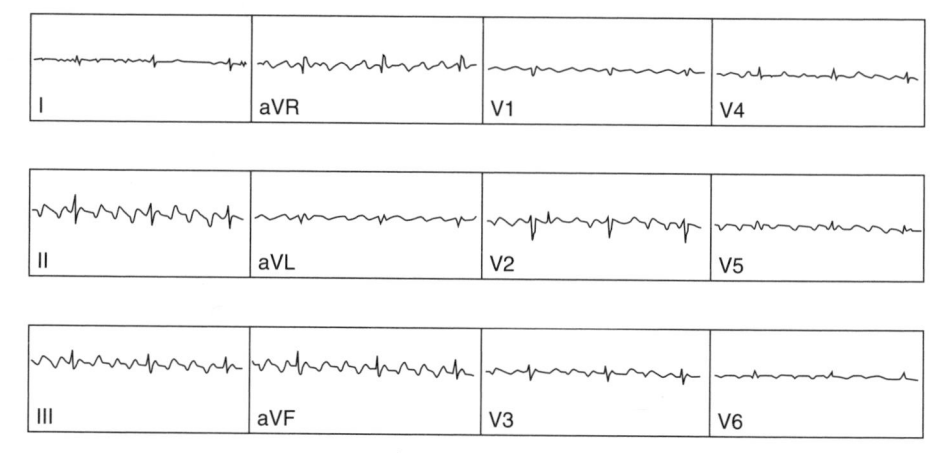

**Figure 10–16** • Typical atrial flutter shown in a 12-lead ECG. Note the sawtooth flutter waves seen in leads II, III, and aVF. This sawtooth pattern is the classic diagnostic feature of typical atrial flutter seen on the surface 12-lead ECG.

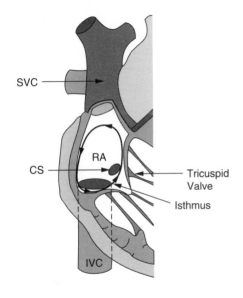

**Figure 10–17** • Typical atrial fluter reentrant circuit. The reentrant wave front travels superiorly along the atrial septum and inferiorly along the lateral atrial wall. The wave front is forced through the inferior vena cava–tricuspid valve isthmus. This isthmus of tissue is a critical part of the reentrant circuit and is the region targeted during radiofrequency catheter ablation. SVC = superior vena cava; CS = coronary sinus; RA = right atrium; IVC = inferior vena cava.

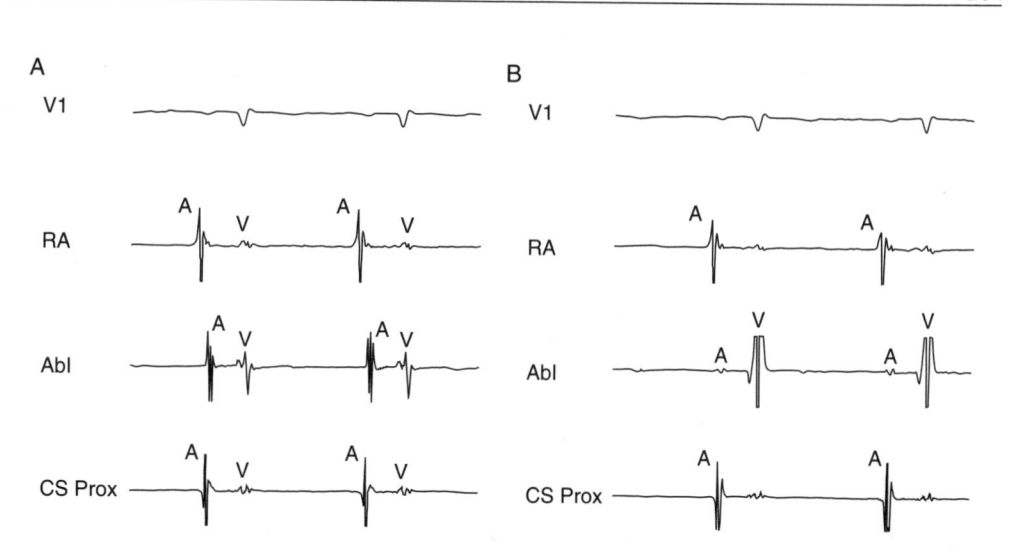

**Figure 10-18** • Atrial flutter ablation sites. **(A, B)** Recordings from surface lead $V_1$ and intracardiac recordings from the right atrium (RA), ablation catheter (Abl), and proximal coronary sinus (CS Prox). Both recordings are made during normal sinus rhythm in a patient who is undergoing ablation of the inferior vena cava tricuspid valve isthmus. **(A)** Note that the atrial electrogram (A) is larger than the ventricular electrogram (V)—on the ablation catheter, indicating that the ablation tip is located proximally in the isthmus region. **(B)** The atrial electrogram (A) is much smaller than the ventricular electrogram (V) on the ablation catheter, indicating that the ablation tip is now advanced much more distally toward the tricuspid valve.

tion catheter is pulled back more proximally toward the inferior vena cava, the atrial electrogram increases and the ventricular electrogram decreases in size.

## Radiofrequency Application

Radiofrequency lesions must be created along the entire continuum of sites between the tricuspid valve and inferior vena cava. A common approach is to deliver the initial RF lesions more distally, near the tricuspid valve, and progressively pull the ablation catheter back more proximally, applying RF current along the way. The RF current is usually applied at power outputs of 25–50 watts or temperature settings of 65°–80°C for 60–90 seconds. If the temperature is not monitored, the impedance should be monitored and the power titrated to achieve an impedance drop of 5–10 ohms to ensure adequate heating. After a complete line of RF lesions has been delivered, the efficacy of the ablation is assessed. If a complete line of conduction block has not been accomplished, repeat ablation lesions are created.

## Determinants of Success

If the patient is in atrial flutter during the RF applications, an initial indicator of success is termination of the atrial flutter (Figure 10–19). A more important endpoint is the creation of a line of conduction block at the inferior vena cava–tricuspid valve isthmus. The advantage of having this endpoint is that patients are not required to be in atrial flutter during the ablation, and creation of a line of block confers a greater long-

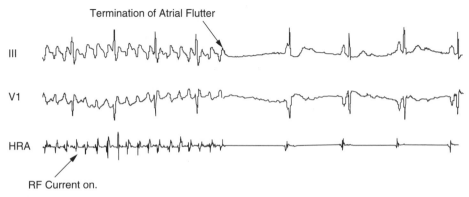

**Figure 10-19 •** Termination of atrial flutter with radiofrequency (RF) current. Recordings from surface leads III and V$_1$ and intracardiac recordings from the high right atrium (HRA) are shown. The ablation catheter was positioned in the inferior vena cava–tricuspid valve isthmus, and the RF current was turned on. The atrial flutter terminated within approximately 2 seconds of the current application, and sinus rhythm was restored. It should be noted that this was not the sole application of RF current but one of the many required to create a complete line of block in the inferior vena cava–tricuspid valve isthmus.

term success than using the inability to induce atrial flutter as an endpoint. A line of conduction block can be evaluated by pacing at different points in the right atrium near the tricuspid annulus and analyzing the spread of conduction around the annulus. A simple method is to pace from the low lateral right atrium and simultaneously record from the His bundle region and proximal coronary sinus. Prior to creating a line of block, the coronary proximal sinus region is activated before the His bundle region, usually with a pacing stimulus-to-proximal coronary sinus atrial electrogram time of 100 ms or less. After creating a line of block there is reversal of the activation sequence, with the His bundle region being activated before the proximal coronary sinus region, and an increase in the pacing stimulus to proximal coronary sinus atrial electrogram time of more than 25 ms from baseline (Figure 10–20). Pacing from the proximal coronary sinus and recording from the low lateral right atrium should also demonstrate a more than 25-ms increase in this conduction time from baseline, indicating that the line of block is bidirectional.

## Complications

The risk of complications is small and primarily related to the risk of catheter-induced trauma during mapping and ablation.

# SINUS NODE MODIFICATION

## Indications

Sinus node function is markedly enhanced in a small group of patients, resulting in chronically elevated heart rates. These patients generally have a baseline sinus tachycardia and an exaggerated response to sympathetic stimulation. In patients who are symptomatic and not responsive to pharmacologic therapy, sinus node modification with RF energy is an alternative approach to therapy.

## Mapping

A combined approach using both anatomic landmarks and activation timing may be appropriate. The sinus node lies in the superior aspect of the right atrium near the right atrial–superior vena cava junction and extends down along the lateral right atrial wall. The most superior medial aspect of the sinus node is responsible for the fastest rates of sinus node discharge. This portion is located near the superior portion of the crista terminalis. The crista terminalis is an anatomic landmark that extends up the lateral right atrial wall and separates the trabeculated atrium from the smooth right atrium (Figure 10–21). Sinus node modification is performed by ablating the sinus node from its most superior site to its more inferior locations in a stepwise fashion. This approach eliminates regions with the fastest discharge rates first; thus the sinus node rate can be titrated downward.

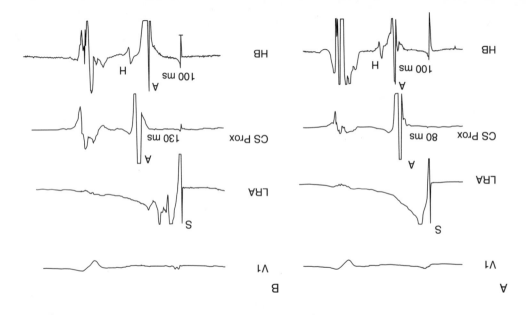

**Figure 10-20** • Pacing technique that can be used to evaluate for a line of conduction block in the inferior vena cava–tricuspid valve isthmus. **(A, B)** Recordings from surface lead $V_1$ and intracardiac recordings from the low lateral right atrium (LRA), proximal coronary sinus (CS prox), and His bundle region (HB). **(A)** Recordings were made prior to the ablation procedure. The low lateral right atrium was paced (S) at a cycle length of 500 ms, and recordings were made from the proximal coronary sinus and His bundle region. The time from the pacing stimulus-to-the atrial electrogram in the proximal coronary sinus was 80 ms, and to the atrial electrogram (A) at the His bundle region it was 100 ms. Note that the atrial electrogram at the proximal coronary sinus occurs before the atrial electrogram at the His bundle region. **(B)** Recorded after creation of a line of conduction block in the inferior vena cava–tricuspid valve isthmus. Again, the low lateral right atrium was paced (S) at a cycle length of 500 ms. The stimulus-to-atrial electrogram time in the proximal coronary sinus is 130 ms, and the stimulus-to-atrial electrogram time at the His bundle region is the same as before ablation at 100 ms. Note also that the atrial electrogram at the His bundle region occurs before the atrial electrogram at the proximal coronary sinus. This increase in the stimulus-to-atrial electrogram time in the proximal coronary artery sinus and the change in the atrial activation sequence is consistent with a line of conduction block in the inferior vena cava–tricuspid isthmus.

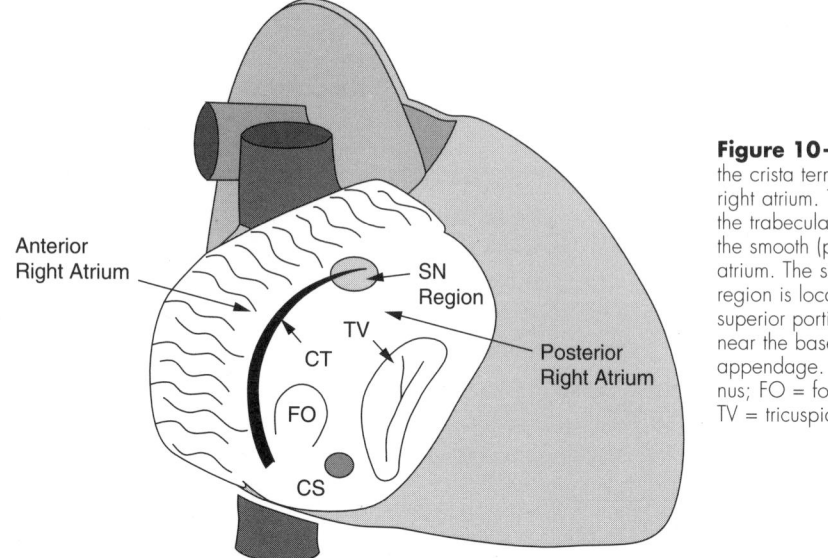

**Figure 10-21 •** Location of the crista terminalis (CT) in the right atrium. The CT separates the trabeculated (anterior) from the smooth (posterior) right atrium. The sinus node (SN) region is located along the superior portion of the CT, near the base of the right atrial appendage. CS = coronary sinus; FO = foramen ovule; TV = tricuspid valve.

The ablation process is started by positioning the ablation catheter in the superior right atrium along its anterior wall using fluoroscopic guidance. The sinus node region is more precisely localized by looking for the area with the earliest atrial electrogram timing. Electrogram timing can be measured relative to the onset of the surface P wave or using a stable intracardiac reference electrogram located in the high right atrium. An alternative approach for localizing the sinus node region is to use intracardiac ultrasonography. This method can identify the crista terminalis, which appears as a ridge of tissue separating the posterior from the anterior right atrium. Intracardiac ultrasonography can be used to guide the ablative tip along the crista terminalis from superior to more inferior locations; its use may improve efficacy and decrease the complications associated with sinus node modification.

## Radiofrequency Application

Radiofrequency energy is usually applied at power outputs of 20–35 watts or temperatures of 60°–80°C for 30–60 seconds. If temperature is not monitored, impedance drops of 5–10 ohms from baseline are generally good indications of adequate heating.

## Determinants of Success

As the sinus node is progressively ablated, the baseline sinus rate and the response to isoproterenol gradually decrease. During the RF applications at regions located along the sinus node, an initial sinus tachycardia is often seen followed by a decrease in the sinus rate. This initial sinus tachycardia is a good indicator that the sinus node region is being affected. Reasonable endpoints for ablations are the creation of baseline sinus rates of 60–80 bpm with heart rates during an isoproterenol infusion (2 mg/min) of 100–120 bpm.

## Complications

The most common complication is the creation of inappropriate sinus bradycardia and sinus pauses. Patients may develop significant sinus bradycardia or sinus pauses up to 24–48 hours after the ablation procedure and should be monitored for this time. Bradycardia requiring pacemaker placement is estimated to occur in 10–15% of cases. This complication may be decreased by the use of intracardiac ultrasonography.

## VENTRICULAR TACHYCARDIA ABLATION

### Indications

There are many clinical subtypes of ventricular tachycardia, but only a select few of them are amenable to treatment with RF catheter ablation. Patients with ventricular tachycardia not associated with underlying heart disease ("idiopathic ventricular tachycardia") comprise the subgroup for which RF ablation has been used most successfully. In this group, curative therapy with success rates of approximately 90%, similar to those for treating paroxysmal supraventricular tachycardia, have been achieved. These patients usually have ventricular tachycardia that is not life-threatening and arises from either the right ventricular outflow tract or inferoseptal region of the left ventricle. Bundle branch reentrant ventricular tachycardia, which usually occurs in patients with dilated cardiomyopathies, is also curable with a high success rate ($\geq 95\%$) using RF ablation. These patients, because of associated heart disease, may have other forms of ventricular tachycardia; and the decision to perform ablation should be guided by whether alternative therapy for other associated ventricular tachycardias is required.

The largest patient group with ventricular tachycardia includes those with underlying coronary artery disease. Within this group only a small number of patients are considered good candidates for catheter ablation. Patients who are considered the best candidates are those with frequent or incessant monomorphic ventricular tachycardia that is hemodynamically stable. In these highly selected patients, RF ablation has an efficacy of approximately 70%. Ablation is usually used as adjunctive therapy in combination with antiarrhythmic drugs or an implantable defibrillator, as these patients almost universally have other forms of ventricular tachycardia in addition to the one targeted for ablation.

## Mapping

The specific mapping techniques that can be used during the ablation procedure depends on the clinical subtype of ventricular tachycardia being targeted. In this section we describe the various mapping approaches and discuss the types of ventricular tachycardia that can be approached using each.

## Pace Mapping

Conceptually, pace mapping is probably the easiest approach to understand and can be used with almost any type of ventricular tachycardia. It is most useful for idiopathic ventricular tachycardias especially those arising from the right ventricular outflow tract. With this technique, a 12-lead ECG of the ventricular tachycardia is obtained after induction of the tachycardia. The ablation catheter is then moved to different locations in either the right or left ventricle depending on the chamber from which the tachycardia originates. At the various mapping locations, pacing is performed from the distal tip of the ablation catheter at a rate similar to the ventricular tachycardia rate, and a 12-lead ECG is obtained. A lead-by-lead comparison is then made between the 12-lead ECG obtained during ventricular tachycardia and that obtained during pacing (Figure 10–22). If the QRS configurations during pacing match the ventricular tachycardia QRS configurations nearly identically in 10 or more leads, the pace map is considered adequate and has identified an appropriate spot for RF application.

## Activation Mapping

Activation mapping is performed with the patient in ventricular tachycardia. Therefore the tachycardia should be hemodynamically stable. With the patient in tachycardia, the ablation catheter is moved to various locations in either the right or left ventricle. The electrograms recorded from the distal electrode pair of the ablation catheter are analyzed and timed relative to the onset of the QRS complex (Figure 10–23). In patients with coronary artery disease-related ventricular tachycardia, activation times of 70 ms or more before the onset of the surface QRS are considered relatively early, whereas in patients with idiopathic ventricular tachycardia activation times of more than 40 ms before the QRS onset are rarely seen. Unfortunately, there is no specific activation time indicative of a successful ablation site, which limits the utility of this approach.

## Mid-diastolic Potentials

This mapping technique is useful in patients with reentrant ventricular tachycardias when there is activation of a critical slow zone of conduction in the reentrant circuit during electrical diastole (Figure 10–24). It is primarily used in patients with coronary artery disease. As with activation mapping, patients must be in tachycardia during the mapping, so their tachycardia must be well tolerated. During tachycardia the ablation catheter is moved to various locations in the ventricle. The local electrograms from the distal electrode pair of the catheter are recorded and analyzed for the presence of electrical activity during diastole. These electrical potentials are often small, and high gain settings on the ablation catheter recordings are usually required. Isolated mid-diastolic potentials are discrete electrical signals seen in the midportion of electrical diastole and are separated from the major ventricular electrogram by an isoelectric interval (Figure 10–25). These electrical signals are thought to represent activation of the critical slow zone of conduction in the reentrant circuit and are acceptable sites for RF application. It is also possible that these mid-diastolic potentials are the result of activation of slow zones that are not a critical part of the ventricular tachycardia circuit (Figure 10–24). Pacing maneuvers at the mapping sites can sometimes be helpful for differentiating critical from noncritical zones of slow conduction.

A

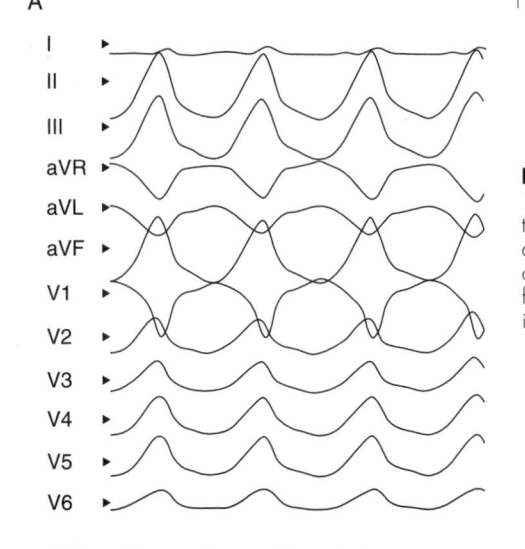

I

II

III

aVR

aVL

aVF

V1

V2

V3

V4

V5

V6

**Figure 10-22 •** Pace mapping. **(A, B)** Surface 12-lead ECGs. **(A)** Recorded during ventricular tachycardia with a cycle length of 320 ms. This arrhythmia was an idiopathic ventricular tachycardia originating from the right ventricular outflow tract and had the characteristic left bundle inferior axis morphology.

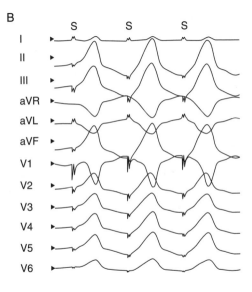

**Figure 10-22 • (B)** Recorded during pacing (S) at a cycle length of 320 ms from the tip of the ablation catheter at a location in the right ventricular outflow tract. The morphology of the paced QRS complex matched the morphology of the ventricular tachycardia QRS complex nearly identically in each lead. Radiofrequency ablation at this location resulted in elimination of the tachycardia.

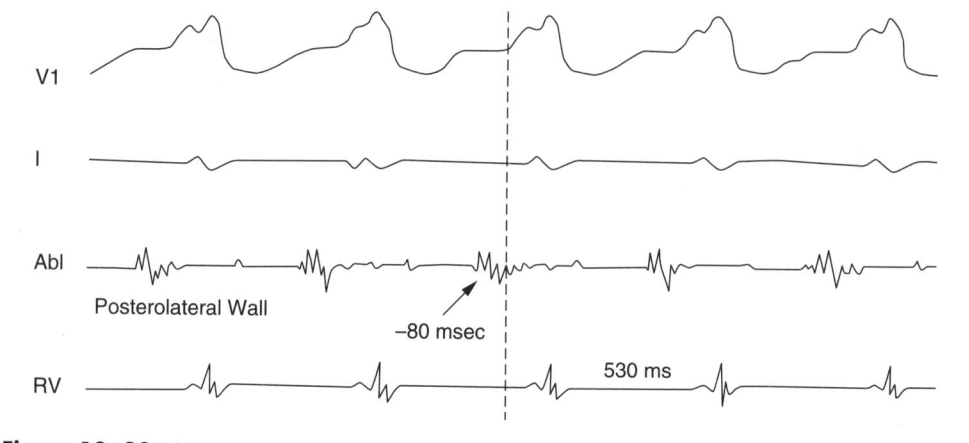

**Figure 10-23** • Activation mapping. These recordings were made from a patient with an ischemic cardiomyopathy and recurrent monomorphic ventricular tachycardia. Shown are recordings from surface leads $V_1$ and I and intracardiac recordings from the ablation catheter (Abl) located along the posterolateral left ventricles and right ventricle (RV). The patient was in ventricular tachycardia with a cycle length of 530 ms. A site was found with presystolic electrical activity, and an activation time of −80 ms was measured relative to the onset of the QRS complex. Radiofrequency application at this site resulted in termination of the ventricular tachycardia.

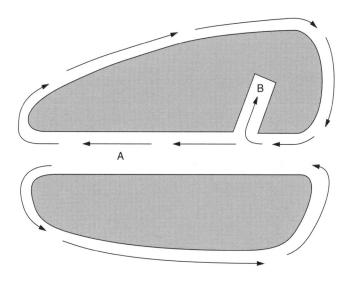

**Figure 10-24** • Ventricular tachycardia reentrant circuit. A proposed reentrant circuit is shown for a patient with coronary artery disease-related ventricular tachycardia (VT). The VT wavefront travels through a zone of slow conduction (A) during electrical diastole. This region is bounded by areas of functional and anatomic conduction block (darkened areas). At the end of the slow zone the wavefront emerges to excite the bulk of the ventricular myocardium and then reenters the slow zone to complete the circuit and sustain the tachycardia. Note that there can be areas of slow conduction (B) that are not critical to the reentrant circuit but attach to the critical slow zone (A).

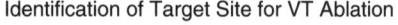

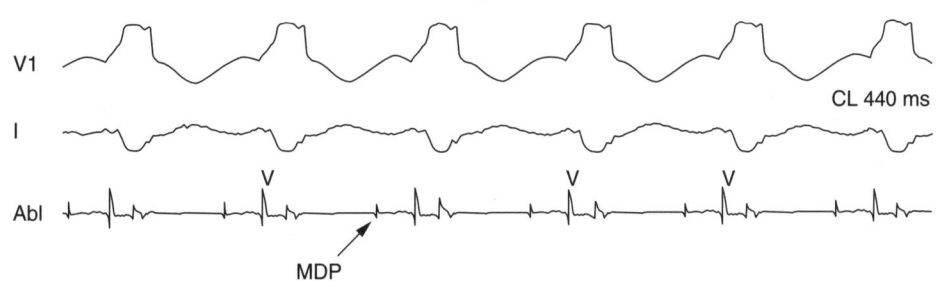

**Figure 10-25 •** Mid-diastolic potential. Recordings from surface leads V₁ and I and intracardiac recordings from the ablation catheter (Abl), located along the inferior wall of the left ventricles, are shown. At this location there was an isolated mid-diastolic potential (MDP) that was separated from the major ventricular electrogram (V) by intervening isoelectric intervals. CL = cycle length.

## Concealed Entrainment

Concealed entrainment is said to occur when pacing is performed during ventricular tachycardia at rates faster than the tachycardia rate and the tachycardia is accelerated to the pacing rate without any change in QRS morphology (Figure 10–26). This situation can occur when pacing is performed at sites within the critical slow zone of the reentrant circuit. During pacing at these sites, there is usually a long pacing stimulus-to-QRS interval because the impulse is traveling through a zone of slow conduction. When a mapping location is found with an early activation time or mid-diastolic potential, pacing is performed to look for concealed entrainment. If concealed entrainment is seen, this area is considered a good target site for ablation. If the pacing stimulus-to-QRS complex time during concealed entrainment is the same as the activation time or the time from the mid-diastolic potential to the QRS complex, it is further evidence that this is a part of the critical slow zone and an excellent site for RF application.

## Purkinje Potential Mapping

Purkinje potential mapping is utilized in patients with idiopathic ventricular tachycardia arising from the inferoseptal region of the left ventricle. This tachycardia, with a typical right bundle branch block/left anterior hemiblock morphology, is thought to be due to reentry that involves a portion of the left posterior fascicle (Figure 10–27). When patients are diagnosed with idiopathic left ventricular tachycardia, the inferoseptal region of the left ventricle is mapped during tachycardia to locate discrete sharp potentials that occur just before the onset of the local ventricular electrogram. These potentials are thought to represent

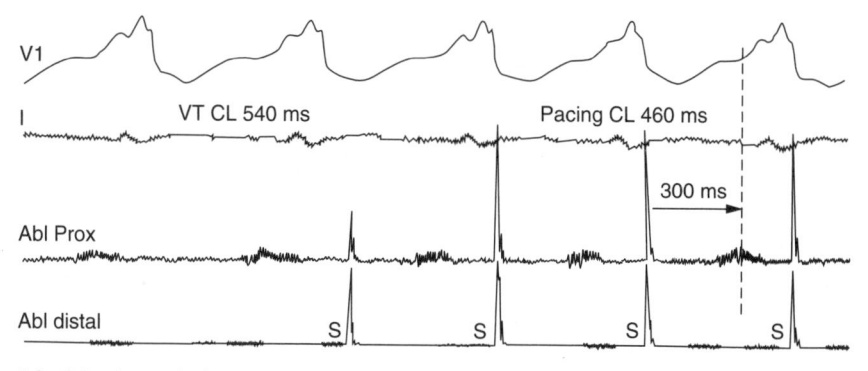

**Figure 10–26 •** Concealed entrainment. Shown are recordings from surface leads V₁ and I and intracardiac recordings from the proximal and distal electrode pair of the ablation catheter (Abl Prox, Abl distal) located along the posterolateral left ventricle. Pacing was performed from the distal electrode pair of the ablation catheter, and therefore no electrograms could be seen on this catheter. The ventricular tachycardia (VT) had a cycle length of 540 ms, and pacing was performed at a cycle length of 460 ms. The pacing accelerated the tachycardia to the pacing cycle length with no change in the morphology of the QRS complexes. Note also there was a long stimulus (S)-to-QRS onset (300 ms). These features are consistent with concealed entrainment and indicate that the catheter is located at a site appropriate for radiofrequency ablation.

activation of the Purkinje fibers from the left posterior fascicle, which are critical to the reentrant circuit. The best ablation locations are those with the earliest occurring Purkinje potentials (Figure 10–28).

## Bundle Branch Mapping

Bundle branch mapping is used in patients with bundle branch reentrant ventricular tachycardia. This tachycardia typically occurs in patients with dilated cardiomyopathies, either ischemic or nonischemic, and associated His-Purkinje system disease. The tachycardia usually has a left bundle superior axis morphology and is the result of reentry between the right and left bundle branches. Ablation of either limb of the reentrant circuit can effectively cure the tachycardia; however, the right bundle branch is typically easier to ablate than the left bundle branch. The right bundle potential is easily localized by first finding the His bundle potential and advancing the catheter farther into the right ventricle along the His-Purkinje axis until the atrial electrogram becomes small or disappears completely (Figure 10–29). Mapping can be done with the patient in sinus rhythm or during tachycardia. Once the right bundle has been localized, RF energy is applied.

## Radiofrequency Application

The techniques for RF energy application depend on the type of ventricular tachycardia being ablated. In patients with tachycardias arising from the left ventricle where coagulum formation is more of a concern

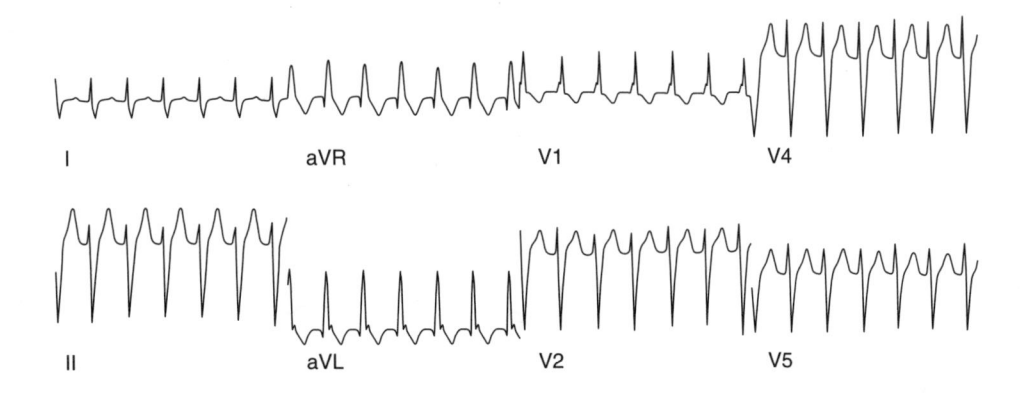

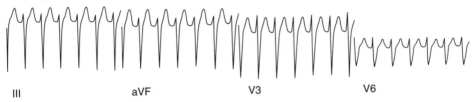

| | | | |
|---|---|---|---|
| III | aVF | V3 | V6 |

**Figure 10-27 •** Idiopathic left ventricular tachycardia. This 12-lead ECG is from a patient with idiopathic ventricular tachycardia that arose from the inferoseptal region of the left ventricle. The tachycardia was thought to be due to reentry involving a portion of the left posterior fascicle. Note the right bundle branch superior axis morphology, which is characteristic of this tachycardia.

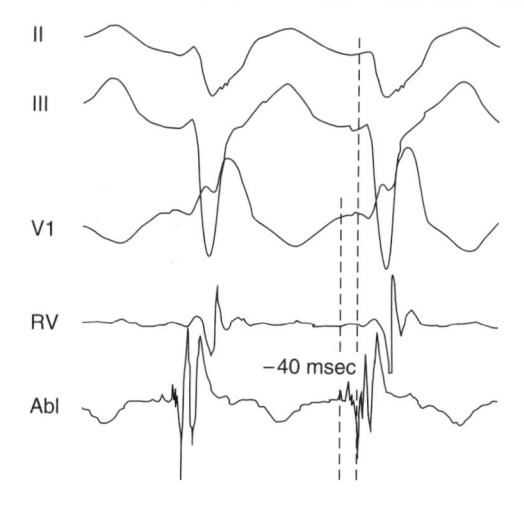

II

III

V1

RV

−40 msec

Abl

**Figure 10–28 •** Purkinje potential mapping. Shown are recordings from surface leads II, III, and $V_1$ and intracardiac recordings from the right ventricle (RV) and ablation catheter (Abl). An electrical potential was found that occurred 40 ms before the onset of the QRS complex. In sinus rhythm this location recorded a potential consistent with activation of a branch of the left posterior fascicle. Radiofrequency ablation at the site resulted in cure of the tachycardia.

and tissue contact may be problematic, the use of temperature monitoring can be helpful. Temperature settings of 65°–80°C are desired to ensure adequate heating and to minimize the risk of clot formation. In patients with tachycardias arising from the right ventricle, there is less concern about thromboembolic events, and temperature monitoring is not as critical. In these patients either temperature or impedance monitoring can be used, and RF current is typically applied at power outputs of 25–35 watts or temperatures of 65°–80°C for 30–60 seconds.

## Determinants of Success

The primary determinant of success in patients with ventricular tachycardia is the inability to reinduce the tachycardia after RF ablation. In patients who are in ventricular tachycardia during the ablation, termination of the tachycardia with the RF current application is encouraging (Figure 10–30) but does not necessarily guarantee lack of inducibility and long-term success.

Some patients with idiopathic ventricular tachycardia arising from the right ventricular outflow tract have frequent premature ventricular contractions (PVCs) of the same morphology as their tachycardia. In these patients, a reasonable surrogate endpoint is elimination of these PVCs, especially if the tachycardia was difficult to initiate reproducibly. For patients undergoing ablation of the right bundle branch for treatment of bundle branch reentrant ventricular tachycardia, an adequate endpoint is the creation of complete right bundle branch block using the standard ECG criterion.

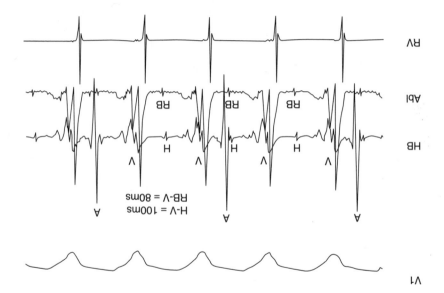

**Figure 10-29** • Bundle branch reentry. These recordings are from a patient with bundle branch reentrant ventricular tachycardia. Shown are a recording from surface lead $V_1$ and intracardiac recordings from the His bundle region (HB), ablation catheter (Abl) located at the right bundle branch, and right ventricle (RV). Note on the His bundle recordings that there are large atrial electrograms (A), and AV dissociation is present. No atrial electrogram is recorded on the ablation catheter, indicating that the catheter has been advanced far enough into the right ventricle to record the right bundle branch potential (RB). The HV and RB-V intervals were both prolonged at 100 and 80 ms, respectively. Radiofrequency application at the right bundle branch site resulted in cure of the tachycardia and creation of complete right bundle branch block.

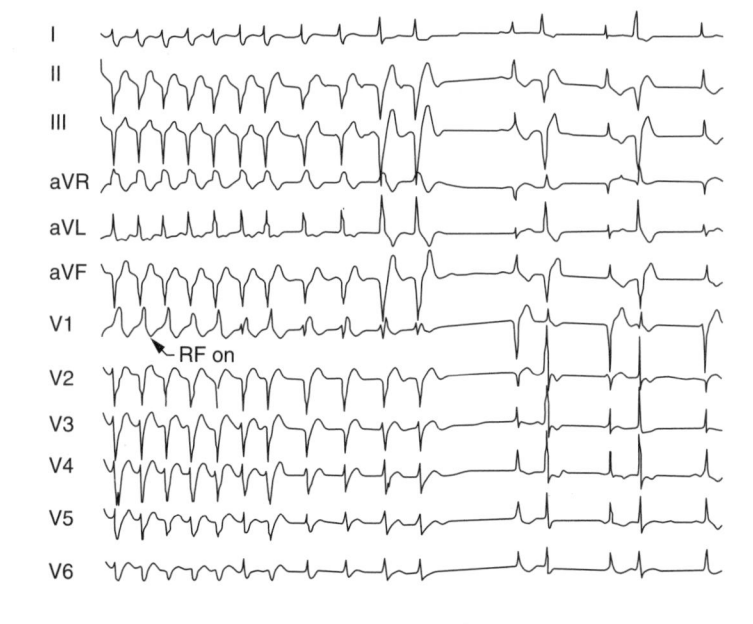

**Figure 10-30** • Ventricular tachycardia termination with radiofrequency ablation. This 12-lead ECG is from a patient with idiopathic left ventricular tachycardia recorded during radiofrequency (RF) ablation. The RF application was delivered at the ablation site shown in Figure 10-28. After the RF current was turned on, the tachycardia began to slow and subsequently terminated. Although encouraging, ventricular tachycardia termination with RF application does not guarantee long-term success, and repeated attempts at re-induction of the tachycardia are necessary to determine whether the ablation has been truly successful.

## Complications

In patients undergoing ablation in the left ventricle, the most significant complications are those related to thromboembolic events or catheter-induced trauma of cardiac structures such as the aortic valve and coronary arteries. These complications are fortunately rare and are generally reported to occur in fewer than 2% of patients. For right ventricular ablations, the most worrisome complication is cardiac perforation and resultant tamponade. Fortunately, this occurrence is also uncommon when care is taken to avoid excessive catheter tip pressure against the right ventricle during mapping and ablation.

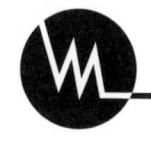

# CHAPTER 11

# PERMANENT PACEMAKERS

Whether permanent pacemaker implantation is indicated in a patient with a slow heartbeat generally comes down to one distinguishing feature of the patient's history: the presence or absence of symptoms. Indications for pacemaker implantation are divided into three classes: class 1, in which the need for a pacemaker is unequivocal; class 2, in which the need for a pacemaker is decided on an individual basis; and class 3, in which the need for a pacemaker is clearly not present. If a patient has symptoms in the setting of a slow heartbeat that is not due to a reversible cause, it generally amounts to a class 1 indication. Class 2 indications usually apply to situations in which the patient has symptoms that seem to be caused by a slow heartbeat but in whom documentation of an event is difficult. Another common class 2 indication is a situation in which the asymptomatic patient's risk of progression to symptomatic bradycardia is thought to be unacceptably high. Detailed explanation of all indications for implantation are beyond the scope of this text. A consensus statement regarding guidelines for permanent pacemaker implantation has been published (*Journal of the American College of Cardiology*, vol. 31, 1998) and is virtually all-encompassing. These guidelines are universally accepted, updated on a regular basis, and can be referred to for specific questions.

## BASIC CONCEPTS

### Pacemaker Systems

The term "pacemaker" refers to the pacemaker system, which consists of a pulse generator and one or two pacemaker leads, or to the pulse generator alone. The pulse generator is the unit that contains a lithium iodine battery and the computer hardware and software responsible for the generation or inhibition of electrical pacing impulses. These impulses are sent from the generator, through the pacemaker leads, into contact with and allowing stimulation of the myocardium (Figure 11–1). Pacing systems can be simply divided into two groups: single-chamber or dual-chamber systems. Single-chamber systems use a single lead placed into the atrium or the ventricle, thereby allowing only one chamber of the heart to be paced or sensed. Dual-chamber systems use two leads—one placed in the atrium and the other in the ventricle—which allows pacing and sensing simultaneously in both chambers. Most (95%) leads are endocardial (placed inside the heart chambers), but occasionally pacemaker leads are placed on the outside of the heart (epicardial) requiring open thoracotomy. The leads in current use are generally bipolar and coaxial. "Coaxial" means that each lead contains two silicone- or polyurethane-insulated wires, one surrounded by the other, with each wire terminating in an electrode (Figure 11–2). "Bipolar" means that the distal portion of the lead contains two electrodes separated by 2–3 cm. The most distal of the two electrodes is the stimulating cathodal (negative) tip; the more proximal electrode is the nonstimulating anodal (positive) ring electrode. The term "unipolar" applies when only the stimulating cathode is in an intracardiac position and the anode is at an extracardiac location (Figure 11–3). Because of the large distance between the unipolar anode and cath-

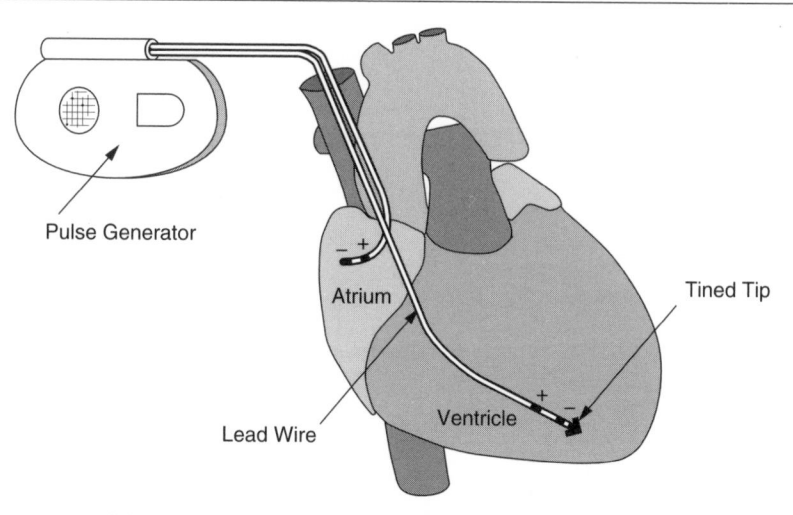

**Figure 11-1** • Dual-chamber pacing system with a pulse generator attached to endocardial pacing leads.

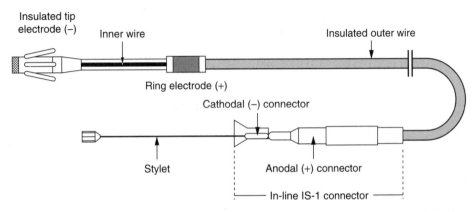

**Figure 11-2** • Bipolar, coaxial lead system. This bipolar lead has closely spaced metal electrodes at the tip end of insulated conducting wires. The lead is coaxial, meaning that the outer wire is wrapped around the inner wire, and they are insulated from each other. The separation between the two distal electrodes is approximately 2–3 cm. The stylet is placed in a central core and is used for shaping the limp lead body.

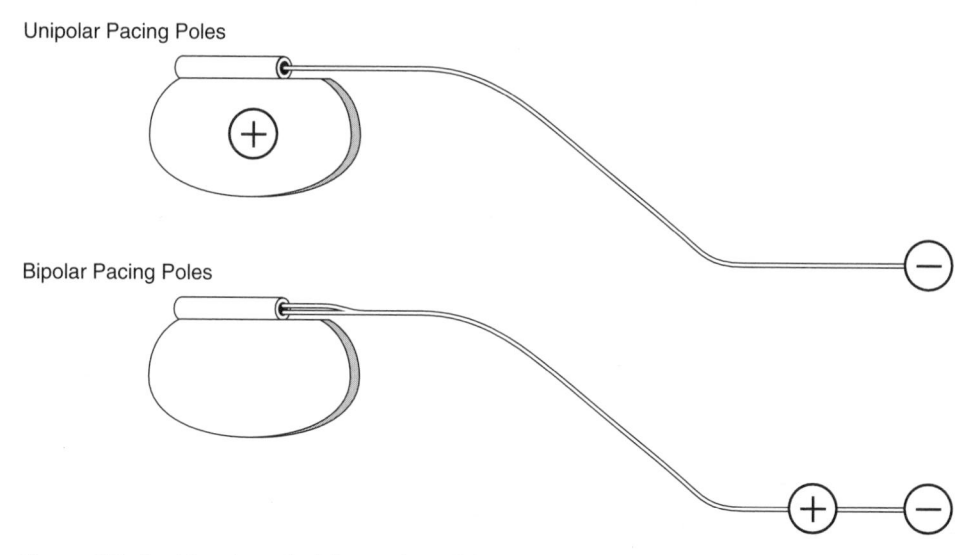

**Figure 11-3** • Note the cathodol (–) and anodal (+) positions on unipolar versus bipolar pacing systems.

ode, pectoral muscle electrical signals (myopotentials) may be sensed by the pacemaker and cause inappropriate pacemaker inhibition (known as myopotential inhibition). Conversely, the pacing output between these two distant electrodes can stimulate the pectoral muscle and cause uncomfortable twitching (Figure 11–4). Except for epicardial systems, which are virtually all unipolar, most new pacing leads currently implanted are bipolar.

The distal stimulating tip is actively or passively fixed to the endocardium. Passive fixation leads have finger-like projections (tines) made of silicone or polyurethane that allow the tip of the lead to catch on the endocardial surface and provide fixation until the lead becomes permanently fixed by fibrous tissue growth (Figure 11–5A). Active fixation leads have a screw at the distal stimulating tip that allows the lead to be actively screwed into the myocardium, providing fixation until the lead is permanently fixed by fibrous tissue growth (Figure 11–5B). Epicardial and endocardial leads can have active or passive fixation.

The lead body is designed to be limp to avoid the risk of perforation and to allow the lead to conform to underlying structures. Each endocardial lead has a hollow core through which a stiff, shapable stylet is placed to allow the lead to be guided into position (Figure 11–2). The stylet is then removed, relieving force at the tip of the lead and allowing the limp body of the lead to conform to the endocardial space.

The proximal connector of currently produced leads is usually a standard IS-1 (3.2 mm) connector: It has two electrodes arranged in an in-line fashion and can fit into the head of any pulse generator with an IS-1 rating (Figure 11–2). Exceptions include older leads, which often have different connector sizes (5 mm, 6 mm), and the recently introduced VDD lead, which incorporates a sensing electrode in a proximal portion of the lead and a sensing/pacing electrode in the distal portion of the lead to allow atrial sens-

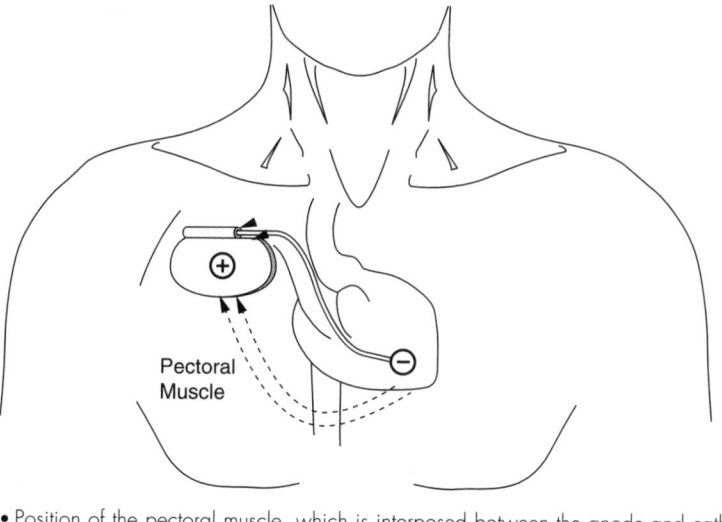

**Figure 11-4** • Position of the pectoral muscle, which is interposed between the anode and cathode of the unipolar electrode. This position allows myopotential detection by the pacemaker with subsequent pacemaker inhibition and pectoral muscle capture during pacemaker output.

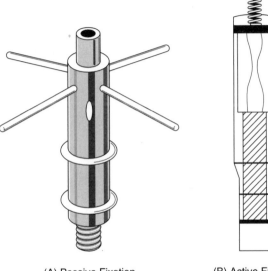

(A) Passive Fixation

(B) Active Fixation

**Figure 11-5 · (A)** Typical passive fixation electrode design with flexible tines projecting from the tip of the lead body. **(B)** Typical active fixation electrode construction with a screw that can be fixed in the myocardium.

ing and synchronized ventricular pacing in a single lead system (Figure 11–6). In both of these examples generator implantation requires a generator with a specially designed lead receptacle (header) or an adapter to allow appropriate contact between the pulse generator and the lead. Before exchanging a pulse generator that is at the end of its life, the exact model of the chronic lead, as well as its size and polarity characteristics, should be known to avoid any lead–pulse generator mismatch.

## Selection of Pacing Mode

Most pulse generators are programmable, allowing selection of different modes of pacing depending on (1) the lead and generator's capabilities and (2) the physician's perception of the patient's needs. The description of the pacing mode is noted by a five-position NBG code that is internationally accepted (Table 11–1). In this code, the first letter describes the chambers paced, the second letter describes the chambers sensed, the third letter describes the response to sensing, the fourth letter describes the programmability of the device, and the fifth letter describes the device's antitachyarrhythmia functions (if any). Thus a pacemaker programmed in the DDDR mode paces dual chambers (atrium and ventricle), senses dual chambers, responds to sensed events in a dual manner (inhibits or triggers), and provides rate modulation. Patients with a VDD lead pace the ventricle but sense both the atrium and ventricle.

Selection of a particular pacing mode is determined by the patient's underlying arrhythmia. In general, single-chamber modes are reserved for patients with chronic atrial fibrillation in whom only single-chamber ventricular pacing can be achieved (chronically fibrillating atria cannot be paced). Single-chamber atrial

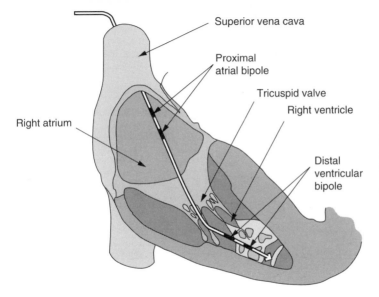

Superior vena cava

Proximal
atrial bipole

Tricuspid valve

Right ventricle

Right atrium

Distal
ventricular
bipole

**Figure 11-6 •** VDD lead with a distal ventricular bipolar electrode in contact with the ventricular endocardium and a free-floating bipolar atrial electrode within the lead body that allows atrial sensing without atrial pacing.

**Table 11-1** NASPE/NBG PACEMAKER CODE

| | |
|---|---|
| I. Chamber(s) paced<br>  V = ventricle<br>  A = atrium<br>  D = double<br>  O = none | IV. Programmability function:<br>  P = programmable<br>  M = multiprogrammable<br>  C = telemetry<br>  R = rate-responsive<br>  O = none |
| II. Chamber(s) sensed<br>  V = ventricle<br>  A = atrium<br>  D = double<br>  O = none | V. Antitachycardia functions<br>  P = antitachycardial pacing<br>  S = shock<br>  D = dual (pace and shock)<br>  O = none |
| III. Response to sensing<br>  T = triggers pacing<br>  I = inhibits pacing<br>  D = triggers and inhibits pacing<br>  O = none | |

pacing can be used for patients with symptomatic sinus bradycardia only in the absence of conduction system disease (which would prevent transmission of a pacing impulse from the atria to the ventricles) and in the absence of paroxysmal atrial arrhythmias (which would prevent atrial pacing). Patients with any significant degree of heart block or with intermittent atrial arrhythmias generally require dual-chamber pacing. Dual-chamber pacing allows restoration of a normal atrioventricular (AV) heartbeat in patients with complete heart block by sensing the atrial beat and triggering an appropriate ventricular output in response (Figure 11–7). It also allows atrial overdrive pacing in patients who develop sinus node disease. Most dual-chamber pacemaker generators can switch from AV pacing to ventricular pacing when atrial arrhythmias are detected, and then restore AV pacing when the arrhythmia resolves (known as automatic mode switching). Clearly, dual-chamber pacing provides the physician with the greatest number of options and therefore is used preferentially when it is not clear how the patient's arrhythmia will behave over time.

Rate-responsive pacing uses a sensor incorporated into the pacemaker generator that allows the device to detect a change in patient motion or respiratory rate. The device then compares the patient's own natural heart rate to what the sensor determines the heart rate should be based on acquired data. If the natural (intrinsic) heart rate is insufficient by sensor criteria, the pacemaker overdrive-paces the patient to provide a faster, more appropriate heart rate to match the patient's level of activity. In a patient who is unable to mount an appropriate heart rate for their activity level (chronotropically incompetent), the rate-responsive feature is often programmed on. Therefore, a patient's pacemaker might be programmed DDDR instead of DDD. Table 11–2 outlines the most commonly used pacing modes for certain underlying arrhythmias.

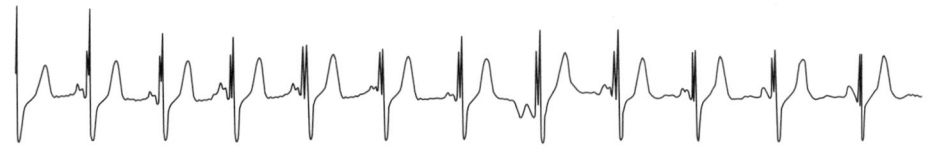

**Figure 11-7 •** ECG tracing reveals intrinsic atrial depolarization with an intrinsic P wave sensed by the dual-chamber pacemaker and a corresponding pacemaker output stimulating the ventricle in response. Normal atrio-ventricular synchrony is restored in the setting of complete heart block.

## Table 11-2 PREFERRED PACING MODES

Sick sinus syndrome:
    DDDR with automatic mode switching
    AAIR if no atrial arrhythmias are present and AV node conduction is intact
    VVIR if patient is in atrial fibrillation
    DDI if atrial arrhythmias are present and mode switching is not available
High-grade AV block
    DDD with rate modulation if sinus node disease is suspected
    VDD when sinus node disease is not present
    VVIR if patient is in atrial fibrillation
Carotid sinus syncope
    DDD with hysteresis
    AAI with intact AV node conduction

See Table 11-1 and text for explanation of the use of letters (e.g., DDDR).

## Electrical Concepts

Pacemaker output pulses can generally be understood through the use of five major concepts: (1) voltage (V)—the force moving current; (2) current (I)—the volume of flow of electricity (measured in amperes); (3) charge—the quantity of electricity that has flowed (amperes × pulse duration); (4) energy—voltage (force) × the charge (measures in joules); and (5) impedance—resistance (R) to the flow of electricity (measured in ohms). Throughout the interaction of all these factors, Ohm's law of electricity applies:

$$\text{Current} = \text{voltage/resistance}$$

The relationship between these various factors determines battery life. For instance, the greater the resistance in a pacemaker lead, the lower is the current drain on the battery: hence the development of pacemaker leads with high impedance to enhance battery longevity.

## Capture and Sensing Thresholds

The *capture threshold* refers to the minimum amount of pulse generator output required to stimulate contraction of the myocardium. Most pacemakers allow the operator to decrease pulse generator output through a decrement in voltage or pulse duration until myocardial stimulation is lost. The voltage or pulse duration is subsequently increased until the minimum amount of energy required to stimulate the myocardium (threshold) is determined. To measure capture thresholds, the pacemaker rate must be set high enough to override the patient's intrinsic heart rate. The capture threshold is usually lowest at implantation and then rises to its highest level (three to four times implant levels) within 2–6 weeks of implantation. The lead then settles down to a chronic threshold that is two to three times the implant threshold. The threshold is measured at the time of implant using a commercially available pacing system analyzer (PSA) that has a constant-voltage power source. These analyzers can also provide information on the current and impedance at threshold. Expected capture thresholds for the atrium and ventricle at implant are as follows:

• Atrium < 1.5 volts at pulse width 0.5 ms
• Ventricle: < 1.0 volt at pulse width 0.5 ms
• Current threshold: 1.5–2.0 mA

The *sensing threshold* determines the pacemaker's capacity to sense the patient's intrinsic heartbeat. The device detects a potential difference between the lead's cathodal and anodal electrodes when the adjacent myocardium is depolarized. This weak electrical signal is detected as the local electrogram by the pulse generator. All recent-generation pulse generators and pacing system analyzers can measure the amplitude (total height of the positive and negative deflections) of the local electrogram, which is expressed in millivolts. The slew rate (rate of change of voltage or slope) of the local electrogram must be sufficiently rapid to trigger a pacemaker. In cases where the adequacy of the electrogram's amplitude is borderline, a sufficient slew rate can ensure good long-term sensing. To measure local electrogram amplitudes, the pacemaker or pacing system analyzer must be set at a rate below the patient's intrinsic rate to allow the patient's intrinsic rhythm to override the pacemaker. Expected sensing thresholds for the atrium and ventricle at implant are as follows.

• Atrium: > 1.5 mV
• Ventricle: > 5.0 mV

## PACEMAKER SYSTEM IMPLANTATION

Most permanent pacemaker implantations are performed using the transvenous approach in an operating room or electrophysiology laboratory. The transthoracic epicardial approach is generally limited to patients requiring permanent pacing who are undergoing thoracotomy for other reasons. This discussion is limited to transvenous implantation. The implant facility should be a sterile environment with appropriate fluoroscopy, electrocardiographic (ECG) monitoring, external pacemaker/defibrillator equipment, oxygen saturation monitoring, and emergent life support equipment. It is preferable that the fluoroscopy table be capable of assuming the Trendelenburg position to increase venous pressure and ease venous access.

Local anesthesia is used for all patients unless contraindicated due to lack of cooperation on the part of the patient. Supplemental sedatives are administered to the patient on an as-needed basis. The wrists are often loosely restrained as a reminder to sedated patients to keep their hands at their sides.

One should always check that there is documentation of normal coagulation status on the patient's chart. An INR in the range of 1.4 with a normal platelet count is generally considered adequate. The site of pulse generator implantation is usually determined by the handedness of the patient and hobbies (e.g., riflery) that would preclude placement near the right or left shoulder. The remainder of this section discusses pacemaker implantation on a step-by-step basis.

## Preparation of the Sterile Field

Ensuring that proper sterile procedures are followed during implantation is one of the most critical steps of the implantation. A sterile surgical approach helps to avoid the catastrophic, highly morbid complication of pacemaker infection. One should be certain that preoperative intravenous antibiotics have been administered.

Preferably, the chest wall is shaved and scrubbed the night before the procedure. If not, it is done prior to sterile skin preparation. The patient's skin in the region of the operative field is then thoroughly prepared with surgical bactericidal solution. At this point, the physician helps drape the field in the usual sterile fashion.

## Formation of the Pacemaker Pocket

When the patient is draped, 1% lidocaine is usually used to achieve local anesthesia using a 22- or 25-gauge needle. Routinely, a 4- to 6-cm incision with a no. 10 or 15 blade is then made approximately 2 cm below the clavicle, beginning at the clavicle's middle third and then drawn laterally (Figure 11–8). If a cephalic approach is being contemplated, the incision is often drawn laterally to the deltopectoral groove. The inci-

251

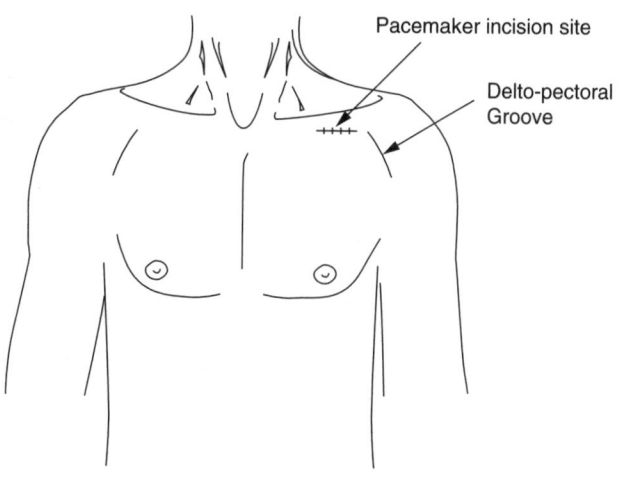

**Figure 11-8** • Incision for pacemaker implantation is performed between the middle third of the clavicle and the deltopectoral groove. It is occasionally extended to the deltopectoral groove for cephalic vein dissection.

sion is then carried down to the prepectoral fascia usually using Bovie electrocautery or Metzenbaum dissecting scissors. At this point, the dissection is taken inferiorly to create a pacemaker pocket in the plane between the prepectoral fascia and the subcutaneous tissue. In extremely thin patients a subpectoral or retromammary pulse generator position may be selected to prevent erosion or to improve the cosmetic result. In the case of subpectoral positioning, higher levels of sedation and a slightly more medial incision are required.

General anesthesia is required for retromammary positioning. A 1- to 2-cm incision is made in the infraclavicular region to gain venous access and allow pectoral lead fixation. An inframammary incision is then made, and the leads are tunneled to a retromammary position where the generator pocket will be located.

Once the pocket is prepared, the operator places an antibiotic-soaked sponge in the pacemaker pocket. One should ensure that the sponge is eventually removed during the procedure, with an accurate sponge count being maintained.

## Approach to Venous Access

Once the pocket is made, attention is directed to gaining venous access, the most common method being the *subclavian approach*. The subclavian vein lies posterior to the clavicle and courses between the first rib and clavicle to join the central venous system (Figure 11–9). It is advisable to have a running intra-

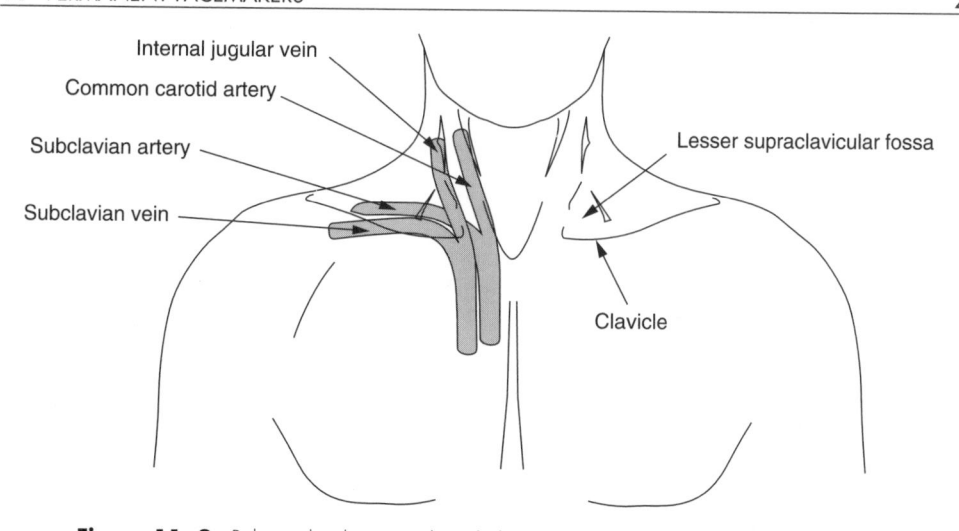

**Figure 11-9** • Relationship between the subclavian vein, internal jugular vein, and clavicle.

venous catheter in the arm on the same side as the venous approach so dye can be infused to ascertain venous patency and guide the needle direction in case venous access is difficult to establish with the introducer needle.

A prepackaged kit containing a needle, guidewire, dilator, and peel-away sheath is then opened (Figure 11–10). One should check with the physician on the desired size (French) of the peel-away sheath prior to opening the kit.

The patient is placed in the Trendelenburg position with the arm positioned straight at his or her side to keep the clavicle aligned. The guidewire is made readily accessible to the operator, and the subclavian vein is punctured with an 18-gauge single-entry needle placed through the infraclavicular incision. The guidewire is then threaded through the needle and passed through the superior vena cava and right atrium into the inferior vena cava under fluoroscopic guidance. Occasionally, the guidewire passes superiorly into the internal jugular vein and must be redirected. In most cases of dual-chamber pacemaker implantation a second needle is used to gain access to the subclavian vein, and a second guidewire is passed. Some operators prefer to retain the guidewire in the venous space after placing the first lead and so use the retained guidewire for introduction of the second peel-away introducer ("retained guidewire approach"). When venous access is established, the pacemaker leads are placed on the table and made readily available.

The dilator is then placed inside the peel-away introducer, and both are passed over the guidewire into the superior vena cava under fluoroscopic guidance. The lead (usually the ventricular lead first) is made readily available, and the dilator and guidewire (unless retained) are removed from within the peel-away

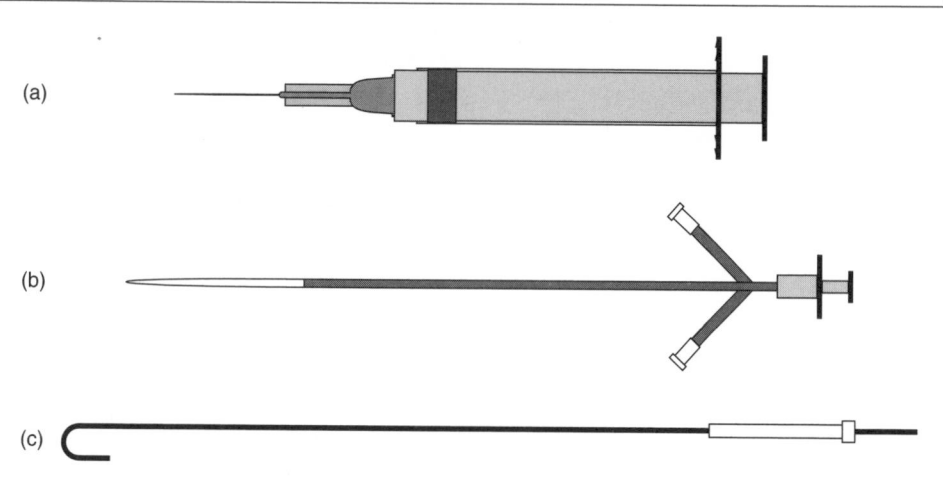

**Figure 11-10 •** Typical introducer prepackaged kit contains a guidewire **(c)**, single-entry needle with syringe **(a)**, and peel-away introducer **(b)**.

introducer, which is pinched tightly to prevent excessive back-bleeding or entrainment of air into the venous space during inhalation. The lead is quickly placed into the central venous system via the peel-away introducer, which is then peeled away.

For dual-chamber systems, a second dilator/sheath unit is placed over the second guidewire (or over the first guidewire if it is retained). The retained guidewire technique allows dual-lead placement with a single needle puncture but increases friction between the leads and decreases their maneuverability. The second lead (usually the atrial lead) is then placed inside the central venous space via the introducer in much the same way as for the first lead.

This subclavian approach cannot be used in all patients. For example, access cannot be established in some cases, and in others the small risk of pneumothorax is unacceptable because of underlying pulmonary disease. Finally, the risk of inadvertent subclavian artery puncture cannot be tolerated by some because of a bleeding diathesis.

For patients with relative contraindications to the subclavian approach, the *cephalic approach* is preferred. The cephalic vein runs in the deltopectoral groove and eventually joins the subclavian vein (Figure 11–11). For this reason, the initial incision is usually extended laterally over the deltopectoral groove to allow dissection. After the local anesthetic is administered, the groove is usually dissected using pickups and a pair of Metzenbaum scissors. Suction is necessary because of the deep location of the vein and should be readily available.

Once the cephalic vein is isolated, a right-angle clamp is used to bring a silk suture around the proximal and distal portions of the exposed vein. The distal suture is then secured around the vein with a knot.

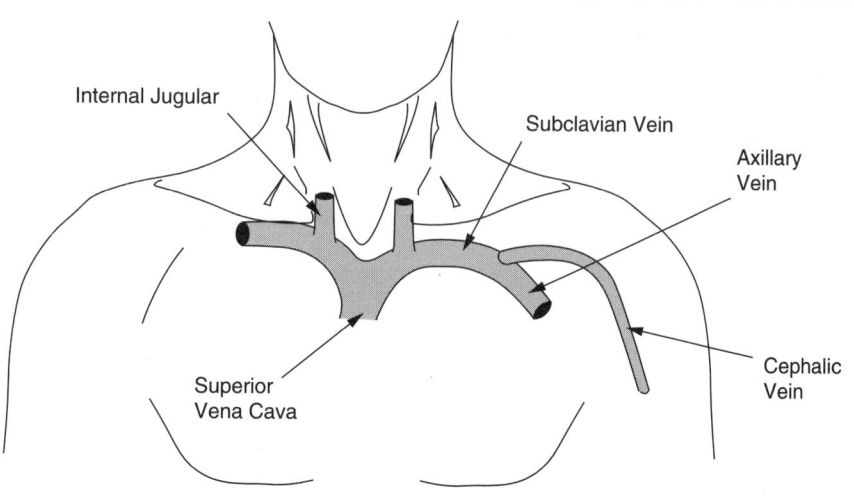

**Figure 11-11** • Relation between the cephalic vein and subclavian vein and the course of the cephalic vein in the deltopectoral groove.

At this point the ventricular lead is opened, as the vein pick in the lead package is needed. A no. 11 blade is then used to make a small incision in the cephalic vein. The vein pick is used to open the incision in the vein to allow the guidewire to be advanced through the incision into the inferior vena cava.

An 11F peel-away introducer is then placed over the guidewire under fluoroscopic guidance. The dilator is removed from the sheath, and the wire is retained within the sheath and clamped to the sterile drape. The sheath is pinched during this maneuver to prevent excessive back-bleeding. The ventricular lead is advanced through the sheath to the inferior vena cava. The peel-away introducer is removed, and another introducer (9F or 11F) is advanced over the retained guidewire under fluoroscopic guidance. The dilator is then removed from the second sheath along with the guidewire, and the atrial lead is advanced through the sheath to the inferior vena cava. The introducer is peeled away.

## Lead Positioning and Testing

Once the leads are within the central venous space they are positioned within their respective chambers for appropriate sensing and pacing. When implanting a dual-chamber pacemaker, the *ventricular lead* is usually the first lead positioned. The straight stylet is removed, and virtually any available tool can be used to form a curve in the stylet. The curved stylet is then placed within the ventricular lead. This stylet curves the ventricular lead, allowing the physician to advance the lead over the tricuspid valve annulus into the right ventricle. The curved stylet is then removed, and a straight stylet is placed into the lead, causing the lead to drop so it can be positioned at the right ventricular apex. At this point the screw mechanism is activated if the lead has active fixation. Figure 11–12 depicts the appropriate ventricular lead appearance.

The lead's sensing and pacing thresholds are now tested using a commercially available pacing system analyzer (PSA). Some operators also want ventricular pacing performed to determine how well the heart conducts impulses retrogradely from the ventricle to the atrium (VA conduction) and to rule out diaphragmatic capture. The operation of each of these analyzers must be taught individually and is not discussed here. The desired ventricular pacing and sensing thresholds are discussed previously. When adequate thresholds are obtained, the lead is sutured to the prepectoral fascia using two sutures around the lead's suture sleeve.

The *atrial lead* is usually placed after the ventricular lead unless one is implanting a single-chamber atrial pacemaker. After the atrial lead is placed in the intravenous space the straight stylet is withdrawn from the lead, and a curved stylet is placed within the body of the lead to bring it toward the atrial appendage. At this point, in active fixation systems the screw is advanced. The lead is tested for appropriate sensing and pacing thresholds using the PSA. When thresholds are adequate, the lead is sewn to the prepectoral fascia using two 2.0 silk sutures. Figure 11–12 depicts the typical appearance of the atrial lead.

## Generator Implantation

The generator is attached to the leads after they are sutured in place. Each lead is placed within the header of the pacemaker, and a wrench is used to fix each lead in position. The wrench is included in the generator kit.

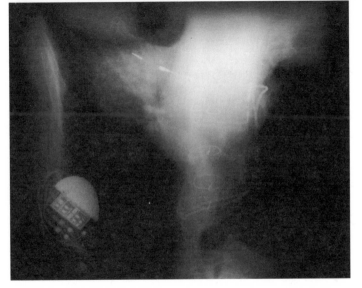

**Figure 11–12 •** Chest radiograph depicts the typical position of the atrial lead (curved upward) and ventricular lead (curved down toward the apex).

The pacemaker pocket is thoroughly flushed with antibiotic solution after any sponges have been removed. The leads are typically pushed into the pocket, and the generator is placed on top of the leads. At this point, an extra suture may be placed through a preformed hole in the head of the pacemaker to allow fixation of the generator to the pectoral muscle, thereby preventing chronic migration of the pacemaker position.

A final check of pacemaker lead position is then performed under fluoroscopy. The pacemaker pocket is closed, typically using a deep layer of suture for the subcutaneous tissue and a layer of fine suture for the subcuticular tissue.

## Pulse Generator Exchange

With appropriate preparation, changing a pulse generator that has reached the end of its life is straightforward. The general considerations and preparation of the sterile field for permanent pacemaker implantation also apply to pulse generator exchange, although the following unique steps must be undertaken prior to a pulse generator exchange.

### Underlying Rhythm Evaluation

When the pulse generator is removed from the lead(s) there is a period when no reliable pacing is available to the patient. Therefore one must determine if the patient is pacemaker-dependent (no underlying rhythm prior to the procedure). Patients who are pacemaker-dependent generally require placement of a temporary pacemaker wire prior to the onset of the procedure. Patients who have an underlying rhythm can generally receive temporary pacing (if needed) via the PSA at the time of pulse generator exchange.

## Chronic Lead Models

Prior to pulse generator exchange the manufacturer and model number of the chronic lead(s) should be known. This information allows one to determine the chronic lead size and polarity in order that a pulse generator with compatible header size and polarity characteristics is available for attachment. Small reference manuals are available from each manufacturer's representative that catalog all lead models and their pulse generator header compatabilities. One manual should be available in each electrophysiology laboratory.

The pulse generator manufacturer's identity is the minimum amount of information required as a starting point. Manufacturers track the implantation of their generators and usually have the lead models at implantation as part of a database that can be accessed. Despite these precautions, unforeseen circumstances may require the use of new leads, lead adapters, or special pulse generators not routinely stocked in the hospital. The presence of the manufacturer's representative at the time of the procedure helps meet any need for unique items.

## Contingency for Lead Replacement

If possible, the chronic pacemaker leads undergo testing for their pacing and sensing thresholds and their impedance prior to pulse generator exchange. This practice allows advance preparation for the replacement of poorly performing leads. Some patients with single-chamber pacing systems require placement of an additional atrial lead, or patients with dual-chamber systems may require only a single-chamber generator and capping of the unused atrial lead. If addition of a lead via the same site is contemplated, intravenous contrast injection on the side of the implantation may be needed to evaluate the patency of the vein to be used for access. If a lead replacement is scheduled, these issues must be addressed with the operator prior to the operation to facilitate the efficiency of the procedure.

## Generator Exchange

Once the general considerations have been addressed and sterile preparation of the field has been performed, generator exchange can be undertaken. Fluoroscopy is often used to visualize the position of the generator in relation to the leads. The pocket is palpated to ascertain that the leads lie below the generator. Local anesthesia is then injected over the site of the pulse generator. Once anesthesia is achieved, an incision is made and carried down, using blunt dissection, to the pacemaker pocket, which is encapsulated in scar.

The fibrous capsule of the pacemaker pocket is then incised with a no. 11 scalpel blade taking care not to damage the chronic leads. The pulse generator and leads are extracted from the pocket and inspected, and the leads are detached from the generator. The pacing systems analyzer is then used to assess pacing lead impedances and the sensing and capture thresholds. The capture thresholds may be much greater and R/P wave amplitudes much smaller than those acceptable at the initial implant. The fact that one is dealing with a chronic lead value, which is unlikely to worsen, allows greater tolerance for "poor" thresholds so long as adequate pacemaker function is not called into question and longevity is not drastically compromised. If the lead parameters are unacceptable, a new lead is placed using the standard implant approaches described previously. If the lead parameters are acceptable, the new pulse generator is attached to the leads. The pocket is then flushed with antibiotic solution, and the scar capsule and soft tissue are closed with a deep suture layer. The skin is closed in the usual fashion.

## Complications

Acute complications from pacemaker implantation occur in approximately 0.5% of cases. The following list details most of the possible acute complications.

- Bleeding
- Pneumothorax
- Cardiac perforation
- Air embolism
- Lead dislodgment
- Arrhythmias

Symptoms such as chest pain and shortness of breath and signs such as hypotension or oxygen desaturation must be monitored throughout the procedure so corrective action can be taken.

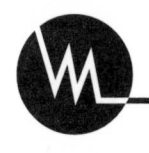

# CHAPTER 12

# IMPLANTABLE CARDIOVERTER DEFIBRILLATORS

Automatic implantable cardioverter/defibrillators (ICDs) were invented by Dr. Michel Mirowski and Dr. Morton Mower to provide an alternative to pharmacologic therapy for the treatment of malignant ventricular arrhythmias. The first human implant was performed via open thoracotomy in 1980 at Johns Hopkins Hospital. Current devices are implanted percutaneously and consist of a generator and a lead system. The generator is responsible for arrhythmia detection, pacing, and shock generation. The lead system allows contact with the myocardium for sensing endocardial signals and delivery of the shock and pacing impulses (Figure 12–1). This chapter reviews indications for implantation, the current systems' features, and implantation techniques.

## INDICATIONS

A joint panel from the North American Society of Pacing and Electrophysiology has issued recommendations regarding indications for ICD implantation (published in the *Journal of the American College of*

*Cardiology*, vol. 31, 1998). These indications were divided into three classes: class 1, general consensus that implantation is considered appropriate; class 2, not a general consensus, but implantation is a therapeutic option; and class 3, general consensus that implantation is not justified. In general, if a patient suffers from a malignant ventricular arrhythmia that is not amenable to pharmacologic therapy, there is a class 1 indication for ICD implantation. Ongoing trials may further expand the next task force's indications to approve ICD implantation over pharmacologic therapy in many situations not previously thought to favor either form of therapy.

## CURRENT ICD GENERATOR FEATURES

The latest-model ICD generators have a lithium iodine battery, capacitors, and the hardware and software necessary to detect the low amplitude, high frequency signals of ventricular fibrillation and deliver several high energy shocks to terminate the arrhythmia (Figure 12–2). These devices also provide backup single- or dual-chamber pacing and the capability to terminate some ventricular arrhythmias with rapid (anti-tachycardia) pacing.

These generators are attached to an ICD lead system. Most lead systems consist of one lead that incorporates a high output shocking coil(s) and a sensing bipole. This lead is positioned in the right ventricle via the right or left subclavian vein.

There has been a marked decrease in the size of the generator, from a volume of approximately 125 cc to less than 40 cc. This evolution in size has changed the implant procedure from one that requires gen-

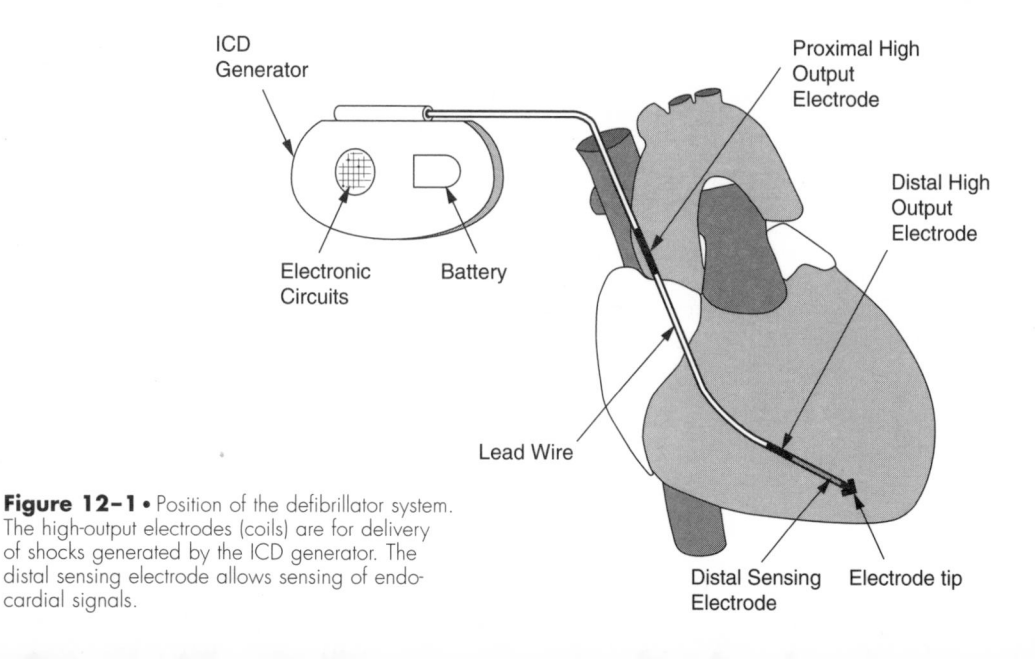

**Figure 12-1** • Position of the defibrillator system. The high-output electrodes (coils) are for delivery of shocks generated by the ICD generator. The distal sensing electrode allows sensing of endocardial signals.

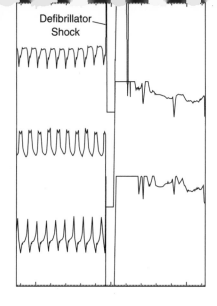

Defibrillator
Shock

**Figure 12-2** • This rhythm strip demonstrates termination of ventricular tachycardia with high output shock from the implantable defibrillator.

eral anesthesia, an abdominal location for the device, and subcutaneous lead tunneling to one that requires local anesthesia, a prepectoral location, and no lead tunneling. Most of the capabilities of the various manufacturers' devices are fairly similar. The following features are those which one must be aware of to work with these generators in the electrophysiology laboratory.

## Detection Criteria

The following criteria are used by the ICD to detect the presence or absence of an arrhythmia.

1. Heart rate: The primary criterion by which a defibrillator detects malignant ventricular arrhythmias is based on the heart rate. The device is set to shock the patient if the heart rate increases above a predetermined level, termed the rate cutoff.

2. Stability: The rate cutoff criterion can be modified by requiring that the arrhythmia not only be fast (above the rate cutoff) but also have regular QRS-QRS intervals by programming a stability criterion "on." The stability criterion requires the heart rate to not change more than a certain percentage from one beat to the next. This criterion helps the device distinguish between ventricular tachycardias (which tend to be regular) and atrial fibrillation (which tends to be irregular with large beat-to-beat rate variation).

3. Onset: The devices can also discern whether a tachycardia starts gradually (as with sinus tachycardia) or abruptly (as with ventricular tachycardia) by activating the onset criterion. This criterion allows

therapy only if the onset of the rapid rhythm is abrupt. Most ICDs can have their detection capability suspended or turned off by placing a ring magnet over the device. If a magnet is placed over the device or is used in close proximity to the device, the device should be interrogated with the programmer to ensure it is still functioning normally.

## Induction Capabilities

All late model ICDs can induce ventricular fibrillation or tachycardia to allow testing of the device's arrhythmia-terminating capability. Each device has different induction algorithms that are usually effective. If the device induction of the ventricular arrhythmia fails, percutaneous catheter placement must be performed to allow arrhythmia induction.

## High-Output Shocking Waveforms

Each defibrillator is designed to deliver a synchronized shock or electrical waveform that converts the heartbeat to a normal rhythm. The most effective shocking waveform is biphasic, in contrast to the monophasic waveform available in first-generation devices (Figure 12–3). The biphasic waveform significantly reduces the energy required to defibrillate the heart, but most defibrillators have the ability to deliver either a monophasic or a biphasic waveform. The shock can be programmed "noncommitted," which means the device "looks" after charging to ensure that the arrhythmia is still present prior to delivering

A. Monophasic Waveform

B. Biphasic Waveform

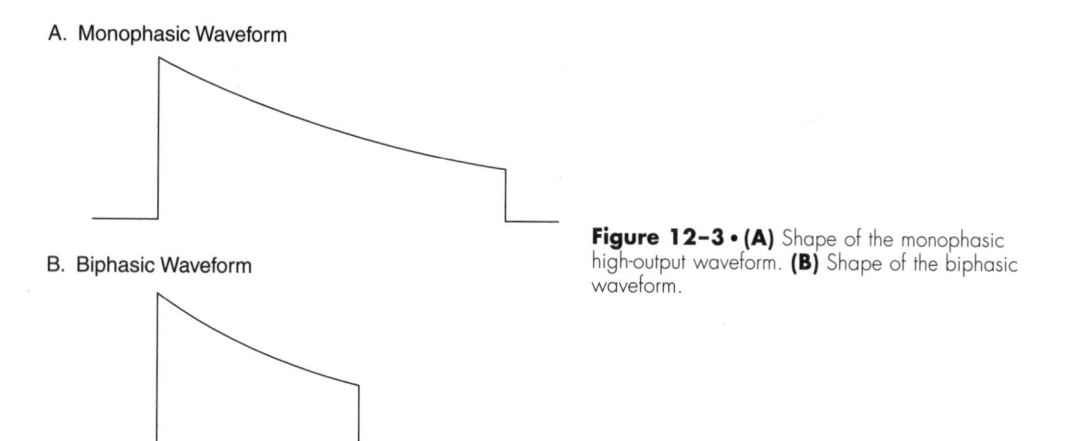

**Figure 12-3 • (A)** Shape of the monophasic high-output waveform. **(B)** Shape of the biphasic waveform.

its shock. Some ICDs allow the physician to program the polarity of the high-output waveform, thereby allowing one to make a proximal or distal shocking electrode positive or negative without manually changing the lead position in the defibrillator header.

## Monitoring Capabilities

All latest-generation defibrillator programmers have the ability to monitor surface electrocardiographic (ECG) activity and intracardiac signals through the device in real time. This ability allows the operator to see exactly what the device sees during sinus rhythm or a ventricular arrhythmia and to correlate it to surface ECG events. The ICD stores intracardiac electrograms preceding, during, and after a shock for the physician to review.

The ICD also stores a record of the number of shocks delivered since the device was implanted and since the patient's last visit. The operator can interrogate lead resistance to evaluate lead integrity and R wave amplitude to evaluate the lead's sensing capability.

## Pacing Capability

All latest-generation devices have demand VVI pacing capability for intermittent bradycardias, which are common after defibrillation. Most of the new devices also have the capability of antitachycardia pacing, which allows termination of ventricular tachycardias via a burst of rapid ventricular pacing (Figure 12–4).

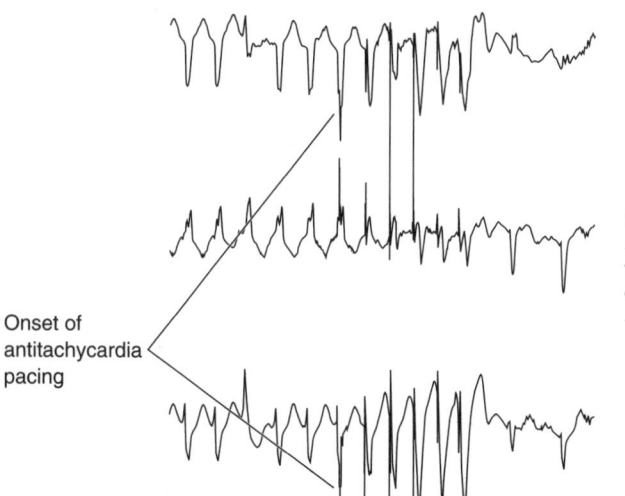

Onset of
antitachycardia
pacing

**Figure 12-4** • This 3-channel rhythm strip was recorded during termination of ventricular tachycardia using overdrive antitachycardia pacing to restore normal sinus rhythm.

Dual-chamber pacemaker/defibrillators are now being released by the U.S. Food and Drug Administration (FDA). They allow dual-chamber pacing and more accurate discrimination between supraventricular and ventricular arrhythmias.

## CURRENT TRANSVENOUS ICD SYSTEMS

Nonthoracotomy defibrillator lead systems are usually implanted via the right or left subclavian or cephalic veins. All ICD leads provide sensing via ring electrodes and high-energy shocks via one or two shocking coils. Some lead systems require placement of two leads. Figure 12–5 shows the structure of a typical ICD lead.

These leads are typically positioned at the right ventricular apex. They can be sutured to the prepectoral fascia and placed in a prepectoral pocket. Alternatively, a longer lead system can be employed that allows tunneling to the abdomen for right or left upper quadrant generator placement. If two shocking coils do not provide an adequate defibrillation energy requirement (evaluated during implantation), a third shocking coil, subcutaneous patch, or subcutaneous array can be added. The "hot can" device allows one to use the casing of the generator as a shocking coil. The newer lead systems in conjunction with a biphasic waveform generator provide 98% likelihood of achieving an appropriate defibrillator energy requirement at implant. Atrial leads for dual-chamber pacemaker defibrillators are standard (IS-1) atrial pacing leads.

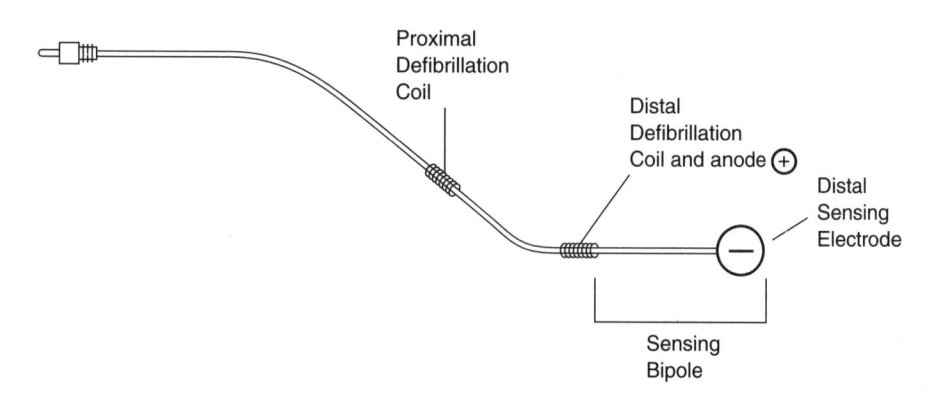

**Figure 12-5** • Typical defibrillator lead. The sensing configuration is integrated bipolar with the distal high-output defibrillation coil as the anodal (+) pole in the sensing bipole.

# IMPLANTATION

Most ICD implantations are now performed using a nonthoracotomy lead system that can be placed prepectorally. Because thoracotomy ICD system implantation represents a small percentage of implants, it is not discussed here.

Equipment required for implantation includes fluoroscopy for nonthoracotomy lead positioning; a pacing system analyzer for lead sensing and pacing threshold determination; an external cardioverter/defibrillator for induction of ventricular fibrillation and delivery of direct current energy through the nonthoracotomy lead for determination of the defibrillator energy requirement (DER) (if one elects to forego device-based testing); an external backup defibrillator; a physiologic recorder for monitoring blood pressure, heart rate, and oxygen saturation; and a fibrillator. A full complement of auxiliary equipment is necessary including lead adapters, subcutaneous patches, and arrays to allow implantation of a device with appropriate energy safety margins.

Necessary personnel include a cardiac electrophysiologist, surgical assistant, and two electrophysiology nurses to monitor patient sedation and operate the external support equipment with or without the aid of an ICD manufacturer's technical support (depending on the level of nursing experience). If an abdominal generator implant is contemplated, it is often necessary to have an anesthesiologist present to provide the appropriate level of sedation for this invasive approach.

The operating room should meet the same sterile standards as for pacemaker insertion. Moreover, strict attention must be paid to sterile technique to avoid the complication of ICD infection.

### Venous Access

The approach to venous access for nonthoracotomy ICD lead implantation is the same as that for pacemaker lead implantation. The only significant difference is that the dilator/sheath size for introduction is usually larger, 11F–14F. Please refer to the section on venous access in Chapter 11 for further details.

### Lead Placement

Every ICD lead system has a sensing lead, which usually has one or two high-output defibrillating coils incorporated into its body. This lead tip is positioned in the right ventricular apex in much the same way as a ventricular pacing lead, as outlined in Chapter 11. Some lead systems require two leads if a second high-output defibrillating coil is required. This lead is usually placed near the junction of the superior vena cava and the innominate vein (Figure 12–6). Each lead is sutured to the prepectoral fascia to prevent it from dislodging. Recent data suggest that it may be best to keep the body of the lead out of contact with the ICD generator, if possible, to prevent lead erosion.

### Generator Placement

Until recently, ICD generator implantation required subpectoral or abdominal implantation to prevent certain erosion because of large generator sizes. Now the device is small enough to be placed prepectorally in a subcutaneous location. After a 5- to 6-cm incision is made infraclavicularly, a pocket is made between the

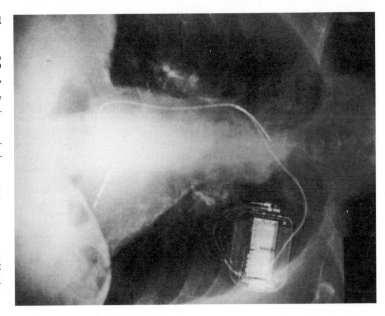

**Figure 12-6** • Radiograph demonstrates proper positioning of the right ventricular sensing/defibrillating lead in the right ventricular apex. There is a separate lead containing the proximal defibrillating coil placed in the superior vena cava.

subcutaneous tissue and the prepectoral fascia. After intravenous lead placement is achieved, the generator is attached to the defibrillator lead pins using the torque wrench, and the device and the leads are implanted in the pocket. An additional suture is often placed through the header of the generator and the underlying pectoral muscle to prevent migration of the device. The subcutaneous tissues are closed usually with a single running suture, and the dermis is closed with a single running suture.

## Intraoperative Testing

A pacing system analyzer is used to evaluate the sensing capability of the ventricular lead. Acceptable sensing and pacing criteria are as follows: R wave $\geq 5.0$ mV; pacing threshold $\leq 1.0$ volt; impedance within the normal range for the lead being tested. These lead parameters often worsen if ventricular fibrillation induction is performed via the pacing bipole, although it is a transient phenomenon.

The energy requirement for defibrillation via the lead system is tested during induction of ventricular fibrillation. An acceptable goal is to have the maximum necessary energy to achieve defibrillation be 10 joules less than the generator's maximum energy output. Alternatively, one may test for defibrillation success with consecutively lower energies until failure, with rescue of the patient via high-energy output from the ICD generator or an external defibrillator. This approach allows the operator to define the minimum defibrillation energy requirement more closely. The device's first shock energy level can then be safely programmed at twice the defibrillation energy requirement. These evaluations of defibrillation energy requirement can be performed through the device after its placement (device-based testing) or through an external cardioverter-defibrillator, which allows such testing prior to opening the new ICD generator (external testing). The pain associated with the induction of ventricular fibrillation and subsequent defibrillation requires sedation similar to that used for cardioversion. Because of the more than 90% success rate with device-based testing, many centers are now adopting this method. External testing is generally reserved for patients in whom high defibrillation energy requirements are suspected preoperatively.

## Complications

Acute complications associated with defibrillator implantation are similar to those seen during permanent pacemaker implantation.

- Pneumothorax
- Lead dislodgment
- Bleeding
- Cardiac perforation
- Arrhythmia

However, because of the greater level of sedation during the defibrillator implantation and the high prevalence of congestive heart failure in these patients, the electrophysiology personnel must be keenly aware of changes in vital signs.

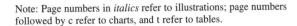

Note: Page numbers in *italics* refer to illustrations; page numbers followed by c refer to charts, and t refer to tables.

## INDEX